Med-Surg RN PRO

The Fearless and Professional Approach to Surviving Your First Year and Beyond of Med-Surg Floor Nursing

Robert McGee Jr. RN, BSN, CMSRN

Table of Contents

Preface 1

Introduction 3

1. The Mindset 7

2. The Preparation 10

3. The Work 18

4. PRO-Insight 22

5. Fighting Your Communication Fears 41

6. Fighting Your Clinical Fears 51

7. Your First Seven Shifts 65

8. Simplifying Weeks 3 - 8 74

9. Managing Months 3-8 84

10. Finishing Insightfully Strong 107

11. Encouragement for the Med-Surg RN PRO 116

Appendices 121

  Appendix A 122

  Appendix B 126

  Appendix C 129

PREFACE

A movement is thrilling. It's the work of many people, all connected, all seeking something better.

Seth Godin

Med-Surg RN PRO is my gift to the profession that has provided me with the flexibility to experience so many precious moments with my beautiful wife and family.

Med-Surg nursing isn't easy or glamorous. It's actually broad and gritty with plenty of room for improvement. I know you've heard the international idiom, "Nurses eat their young." However, the Med-Surg RN PRO movement seeks to change healthcare through a nursing practice that values intentional preparation, healthy work environments, and better nurse and patient care experiences. The habits you form at the start of your career will likely follow you until the end. Your desire to be prepared for your new nursing adventure is awesome and shows that you have massive professional potential. Your habits and how you carry yourself on your floor are the things that your patients, colleagues, and community will always remember about you. I would like to invite anyone who is poised to learn, to lead the movement of leaving Med-Surg nursing better than they found it. If you are now employed or will soon be employed on a Med-Surg unit, you will undoubtedly have an impact on the specialty. In my heart of hearts, I am confident that the person who pursues the goals and mindset of the Med-Surg RN PRO will be a leader of change, professionally and fearlessly. The question at hand is, "What do you want your Medical-Surgical nursing experience and impact to be?"

INTRODUCTION

Congratulations! You've made it to yet another milestone in your nursing journey. I realize this is an exciting time for you and rightfully so. Welcome to the wonderful world of Medical-Surgical nursing. Your first year of nursing will benefit you greatly if you become specialized in **Thinking Forward** and **Figuring It Out**, while understanding the concept of **Task Management**. You are now part of the single largest nursing specialty in the United States.[1] As a Medical-Surgical nurse, you will spend more face-to-face time with patients than any other profession in the hospital.

I've worked on the Med-Surg units as both a staff nurse and charge nurse of large teaching hospitals, as well as a small suburban hospital, since 2012. I've cared for shackled inmates and wealthy executives. One day, I walked on to the unit and was surprised to learn one of my patients was my nurse manager, admitted for a syncopal episode.

---

[1] "About AMSN: What Is Med-Surg Nursing? | Academy of Medical." https://www.amsn.org/about-amsn/what-med-surg-nursing. Accessed 6 Nov. 2021.

I was the favored nurse responsible for caring for my nurse manager for twelve interesting hours. All this to say that as a Certified Medical-Surgical Registered Nurse, I have acquired a great amount of knowledge and experience, and it is my sincere intent to share all of it with you. In writing this, I hope to provide all the wisdom and resources I feel are necessary to help you limit the stress and fear of taking on the challenge of becoming a Med-Surg nurse.

Your nursing school GPA is history. However good or bad, do not allow your GPA to alter your assessment of your ability to successfully transition into the world of Med-Surg nursing. Whether you are working in Med-Surg in order to move on to a more specialized area or planning to become a champion of the Medical-Surgical nursing specialty, this book will offer you insight that typically comes from many years of on-the-job experience.

Med-Surg RN PRO isn't a title you should set out to achieve. The title Med-Surg RN PRO is more of a mindset. Med-Surg RN PRO is the mindset of **Thinking Forward** and using your resources to assist you in **Figuring It Out**. Med-Surg RN PRO is the mindset that will allow you to become the best of the best within the specialty of Medical-Surgical nursing. There will be many demands throughout your shift, but as a Med-Surg RN PRO you will become effective at coordinating your patients' care through seemingly effortless and innovative methods. The Med-Surg RN PRO is the person who is considered an exceptional caregiver, an asset to their organization, and a trustworthy friend to their colleagues.

During our time together, we will identify your goals for your first seven shifts as a Med-Surg nurse. The average new Med-Surg nurse doesn't know what their goals are, but you will. Even better than providing your first seven days of preparation, this book will explore the proper Med-Surg nurse mindset and help you set achievable goals for your entire first year as a Med-Surg nurse. You can, and should, use this book as a classic reference every day for the first year of your Med-Surg nursing journey.

Nursing School + NCLEX + THIS BOOK + 1 Year of High-Quality Bedside Experience = Med-Surg RN PRO.

Becoming a Med-Surg RN PRO is just the beginning of your true nursing life. So, let's get this foundational work out of the way! Let's start your journey of becoming a Med-Surg RN PRO!

1

THE MINDSET

"It's not that I'm so smart. It's just that I stay with problems longer."

Albert Einstein

Figure It Out

There are usually many ways to complete tasks on a Med-Surg unit. The good news is you only need to find one that works. Discovering a way that works best for you is largely dependent on your capacity to **Figure It Out**. What do I mean when I say **Figure It Out**? This is your ability to successfully conquer the challenges before you by utilizing all of your available and thinkable resources. This is the one skill that will separate you from the pack. You will be unstoppable if you learn this skill.

Thinking Forward

Thinking Forward is knowing or considering what your next task will be. As a Med-Surg nurse, you cannot only think of your present tasks. You should habitually think of future tasks and their outcomes. For example, you should start thinking of the discharge plan for your patient the minute they are admitted to your floor. If a patient asks, "What should I expect to happen next?" you should have the answer because you are the nurse who is always **Thinking Forward**. When you can't find the answers, always give your best effort to **Figure It Out.**

Task Management

You will learn and hopefully master the great art of **Task Management**. Research shows our minds can only multitask for automatic behaviors like walking or blinking our eyes.[2] In nursing, you will want to be excellent at focusing your full concentration on one task, then switching to another and then another. Some may call this multitasking, but again, research has proved that there is no such thing as performing more than two activities at the same time with all tasks receiving equal amounts of concentration.

What do I mean by **Task Management?** Safely concentrating on a single task while considering the steps of the next in a way that prepares you to effectively complete an immediate or larger task. As you work the floor, you can expect to always be working on more than one task at a time. Even if you are not physically working on more

---

[2] "The Myth of Multitasking | Psychology Today." 12 May. 2014, https://www.psychologytoday.com/us/blog/creativity-without-borders/201405/the-myth-multitasking. Accessed 6 Nov. 2021.

than one task, your mind should be thinking of the next task on your to-do list. The Med-Surg RN PRO is always thinking one step ahead. **Thinking Forward** is heavily intertwined in **Task Management.**

2

THE PREPARATION

"One important key to success is self-confidence. An important key to self-confidence is preparation."

Arthur Ashe

Safety

Questions are directly tied to safety. Ask questions. The novice nurse who does not ask questions will one day be a very dangerous person. A person who could even face criminal charges. Do not let your shyness or arrogance lead to such a situation. After you find comfort in asking questions, take the next step and seek to ask great questions. It is true that there is no such thing as a dumb question. However, there are good questions, and then there are great questions. The great questions usually involve deep thought.

As a new nurse, you will have many random questions. As time passes, think critically about the questions you are asking. Do not fall into the habit of asking random questions. Your goal should be to ask many great questions. Good questions are usually closed ended questions that newer nurses ask for the sake of removing the awkward silence between them and their preceptor. Great questions are typically open-ended questions that reveal answers in which you could not otherwise find without asking a person who is very familiar with your unit and your hospital's policy.

Throughout your career, you will have a reputation to maintain. Let's call this reputation your "Professional Nurse Brand" or "PRO Nurse Brand." Your PRO Nurse Brand is the unique way that you provide care to your patients. There are many things in life that we have very little control over. Your PRO Nurse Brand is the one thing you have total control over. Pretend you are providing care for your favorite celebrity, and before he/she leaves, they want to speak to the President of your hospital about your exceptional care. This is a huge compliment for you! Pretend this compliment could find its way to your local news media. Take a few minutes to contemplate a few characteristics and qualities that you want this person to mention. Now, keep all those right where they are and move "safe and trustworthy" to the top. Every day or night you walk on to your unit, you have to place the safety of your patients, yourself, and your colleagues at the top of your priority list. Nothing else matters if you are unsafe. Nursing has a way of taking excellent care of you when safety is always your number one priority.

Mistakes

Your PRO Nurse Brand will take many shifts over many years to build, but one mistake can ruin your years of hard work. So, when a mistake does occur, your PRO Nurse Brand will provide a solid base of support for the idea that you may have indeed made a mistake, but that it isn't to be routinely expected. If you are reading this book, there is a good chance you are preparing for success, but you'd be preparing for the wrong thing. In fact, what you should be preparing for is failure. The smart person is training for success, but the smarter person trains for failure. You will make a mistake. However, that mistake should always follow a self-commitment to never make that particular mistake again. This is what makes failure so important. The Med-Surg RN PRO will experience credible successes because he/she is preparing for the possibility of failure. With the proper preparation, you can be sure that failure will not become your identity because you are building a PRO Nurse Brand that should display your prior preparations and a commitment to safe patient care.

If you make a mistake, always make the most of it. Take a moment to reflect on the experience. Evaluating the unintended experience is humbling, but it will bring you a great reward later in your profession. Remember, this is a process that all responsible nurses complete. The humility required for owning your mistakes will lead to the trust of your leaders. Who are your leaders? Your peers who have been nurses for many years, charge nurses, nurse supervisors, nurse educators, and your nurse manager. These are the leaders you will have the most contact with.

You will grow from a novice nurse requiring constant supervision, to self-reflective and trustworthy, allowing more and more autonomy with the goal of you becoming a safe, independent member of your healthcare team. Overlooking the lessons in your mistakes will slow down your progression and require your leaders to blindly guess your commitment to safe patient care based on the mistakes others have experienced or heard about while working alongside you. This could lead to distrust and an unfavorable suspicion regarding the quality of your patient care. Healthcare leaders trust those who have a track record of integrity. Healthcare leaders also know the person who is trustworthy doesn't typically need to be pressured to confess a clinical mistake that could later place the company in unnecessary legal trouble.

Here are a few questions you should ask yourself after a mistake:

- What went wrong?
- Where did it go wrong?
- Why did it go wrong?
- What can I learn from the experience?
- How will I apply what I've learned in the future?

You can actually write out a practical action plan to prevent this mistake from happening again. Once you find a seasoned nurse you trust, ask this person to review your action plan and provide you with helpful feedback. Please don't obsess over the mistake, but it's totally fine to allow another person to know you are serious about limiting the number of mistakes you make. The Med-Surg RN PRO does not end their shift without taking advantage of a significant opportunity to learn. The Med-Surg RN PRO isn't perfect, but he/she is a trusted protector of his/her patient.

Don't Be Too Hard on Yourself

Be patient with the learning curve. Nursing is largely based on taking the critical thinking skills you learn from your clinical experiences and applying them to your current tasks. It takes time to recognize frequent patterns that make you faster and more efficient on the floor. Every time you work you are stacking one shift's experience on top of another shift's experience, which will eventually make you a more efficient member of your healthcare team. You are slowly growing into a critical thinking machine. Oftentimes, the hardest part of being a new nurse is pulling yourself up out of your feelings of frustration and overcoming your insecurities. You're probably doing better than you think. You have to consider all of your previous successes when you aren't enthusiastic about your most recent performances. Please remember, every nurse has been through this process. Never quit on a bad day, and you will be fine. A bad shift does not make you a bad nurse.

Acknowledging your weaknesses is the first step in overcoming them. Here's the reality, there are growing pains in the process of becoming a Med-Surg RN PRO. Understand this, those who take responsibility for making their next decision their best decision, no matter what circumstances life brings them, are much more likely to live out their dreams. Studies consistently show that people who do this tend to outperform those who don't.[3] Be encouraged and don't lose focus of your goals.

Self-Care

Your new position will tire you out, and you may never realize it. A good work-life balance will be imperative. You should start exploring things that relax you. There's a chance you may not know the one thing that is sure to relax you. If this is the case, take some time to try new hobbies. You are looking for your happy place. The one place that takes you away from the cares of this world for a moment. Think about the things you enjoyed as a kid if you can't immediately find an enjoyable hobby. Here are a few activities to consider:

---

[3] "Take Ownership of Your Actions by Taking Responsibility - Harvard ...." 30 Aug. 2012, https://hbr.org/2012/08/take-ownership-of-your-actions. Accessed 6 Nov. 2021.

- Walking by the lake
- Listening to live music
- Fishing
- Poetry
- Going out to eat (alone or with friends or family)
- Running
- Cooking
- Cleaning
- Reading
- Exercising
- Painting
- Attending sporting events
- Crafting
- Volunteering
- Serving at your local church
- Etc.

Your happy place is a crucial aspect of your personal self-care, but the people in your circle are just as important. Effective self-care requires a conscious effort of repositioning the people in your life. At this point in your career, you will need to hear from those who encourage you more than the people who drain you. Allow yourself to be readily available to those who encourage you and challenge you to be your best. Do not confuse this person with the person who creates favorable hypothetical scenarios that conclude with you always being right. You need accountability and encouragement, not an enabler.

Once you have found a hobby and repositioned the people in your life, consider taking a vacation. Did you know you can schedule yourself to have eight days off in a row without using PTO? Pretty awesome right? I will start with a disclaimer; you will have to work three days in a row - twice. Each pay period has two weeks in it (Unless you work for the VA or a government employer with a pay schedule of their likeness). To have eight consecutive days off you will schedule yourself to work the first three days of the first work week and the last three days of the second workweek.

3

THE WORK

"You can't cheat the grind, it knows how much you have invested, it won't give you anything you haven't worked for."

Anonymous

Hard Work

You will work hard as a Med-Surg nurse. There isn't any way around this. Embrace this because being lazy isn't an option. Mentally, you should always assume that every day you put on your scrubs you will hit the ground running. This mentality will create a healthy, task-oriented drive. I say this because laziness is usually the case when someone underestimates the effort it takes to complete the tasks assigned to a Med-Surg nurse. Shortly after the underestimation of their workday and extended conversations, enters a heightened sense of panic. This is generally when the nurse realizes he/she may have wasted valuable time. That poor decision may have cost them their lunch break. Imagine working 13 hours without a lunch break. You can prevent it from happening when you don't underestimate the amount of work required of you as a Med-Surg nurse.

Always remember that money does not reward hard work. Many people sweat a ton and work hard but are paid the lowest wages in their industry. Money rewards those who offer unique value. As a Med-Surg RN PRO, you should be prepared to find solutions to problems that prevent you from working smarter. If you do so frequently, this will be a unique value to your employer and your patients. Search through your daily routine for areas of improvement. How can you become more efficient? After you make adjustments to your routines, you may find that you aren't working harder, but the opposite is true. Your work and days may become easier and more predictable as you make a daily habit of **Figuring it Out** and **Thinking Forward**. If your solution has worked for you, it might help lessen the workload of those around you. Offer your solutions to your colleagues and leadership if they are receptive to feedback from their frontline staff. If not, write down your ideas for the day that you do have leadership who listens. At the very least, your colleagues will value your input and effort to make their workdays easier.

The Med-Surg RN PRO works smarter and offers unique value. You can offer value through an unlimited number of ways in healthcare. You should always be employed if you are a nurse who **Thinks Forward** about the next noble idea, whether it's large or small. When you are continuously thinking of solutions, your total annual income potential will be unlimited. You can very well start your movement inside or outside your organization when you make a habit of **Thinking Forward**. Identify a problem, consider multiple solutions, then brainstorm about the processes and resources needed to reach a measurable outcome for your solution. These are overly simplified steps, but I hope you understand the value you will offer as a Med-Surg RN PRO. Always remember, money rewards those who offer unique value, not those who are busy "working hard."

Communication

Effective communication is an important part of your work. When communicating with your preceptor, patients, family, doctors, or any other interdisciplinary professional, be clear, concise, and speak in simple terms. If your patient or their family member is well educated, they will ask questions that will prompt you to respond with more detailed answers and maybe even require the use of medical terminology. Simple answers with a confirmation from the recipient of understanding are usually enough. You can save the medical jargon for your fellow nurses and physicians.

You are the channel in which information flows from the physician to the patient. Advise your patients early in the shift that you are waiting on their physician to give you the plan for the day. Be sure to communicate to your patient that whenever you hear what the next steps in their plan of care are, you will let them know. Reasonable patients will not become upset as long as they notice you are working towards the next step of their care. Are there any procedures, new medications, consults, surgeries, discharge plans, diet modifications, etc.?

Teamwork

There is freedom as a nurse, but never forget you are an essential part of a team. You may work with a colleague who's an introvert and doesn't talk as much compared to others. You may run across a colleague whose personality doesn't mesh well with yours. This is fine. You can maintain a healthy relationship with these individuals. Never shut down your interactions because of these types of behaviors. I would like to encourage you never to adopt the mindset of working alone. You will see others try to do this. It usually leads to a toxic work environment and decreases the quality of care your unit as a team will provide. The people who don't talk to each other will only talk when a patient is sick, or if there is a legitimate emergency, but even then, their communication is usually the minimum required effort. This behavior isn't a characteristic of the Med-Surg RN PRO. The Med-Surg RN PRO aims to communicate with both our patients and work colleagues effectively. Your patients' lives and clinical outcomes depend on your ability to effectively communicate. You cannot provide high quality healthcare in isolation.

4

PRO-INSIGHT

"Insight essentially means being able to see things other people are not able to see. This is the hallmark of leadership."

Jaggi Vasudev

Time Management

After gathering your morning reports, you should be **Thinking Forward** to plan out your day. Organize your pockets and get busy. The word busy can be deceptive. I will correct myself here. Don't be busy. You can look like you are working hard on the floor and not do one beneficial thing for two hours, especially as a new nurse. Be wise, and use your energy purposefully. Be intentional about completing your next task. After one task, head straight to the next with minimal interruption. The best Med-Surg nurses perfect their skill of **Thinking Forward** about the things they may need the next time they go into their patient's room.

Nurses who plan and **Think Forward** have less stress. Start a running list of all the tasks you need to get done and estimate the time you think it will take to complete the task. Be flexible with this list. Look over your list and address the highest priority tasks first. Whenever you have downtime, you should be **Thinking Forward** about what you will check off next on your list. Don't assume you will have time. If you can complete the task, complete the task. Also, understand that there will be another task that makes its way onto your list soon. Consistently completing tasks is a sure way to relieve stress. Do not let excessive side conversations with patients or other nurses disrupt your workflow. The best time to converse is when the majority of your identified tasks are complete. Don't forget to look over your list and identify which tasks can be delegated.

Time is every human's most valuable asset. You will not get time on your floor back. Place the largest and most dreadful task on your list as a high priority. Don't overthink all the tasks that are piling up. You will have plenty of time to get things done. Just get to work. You will be there caring for your patients for 12 hours. Take your day one hour at a time, have measurable goals for your tasks at that hour mark, and as you complete your tasks, chart your work.

Admit when you are too far behind. This shows that you are self-aware and honest. If you are behind, it's okay to ask your charge RN to complete one or two simple tasks for you. Do this as early as possible, but try not to make this a habit every shift.

Superior time management involves learning how to effectively cluster care. What is clustering care? Clustered care is basically grouping several patient care tasks for a one time patient encounter. It is an efficient method of finding the smartest way to use your time. It involves grouping your tasks to achieve the goal of less stress and higher productivity.

Note Taking

I can guarantee you two things:

1. Your first year of Med-Surg nursing will be a challenge.
2. Your consistency in writing learned information will significantly affect how challenging your first year will be.

While on orientation, you should be writing most of the information that your preceptor is teaching you. Your preceptor does not want to continue to review the steps of a procedure that you have performed many times but cannot remember. Notetaking will impress your preceptor.

I recommend you having a specific area on your nurse report sheet where you make notes. Ideally, you should write these notes down throughout your day and later transfer those notes to a small booklet or note-card. The transfer can occur later that night or the next morning.

This small booklet or note-card will be a lifesaver when you are finished with orientation and on your own as a new nurse.

Examples of things to take notes on:

- Procedures (blood transfusion steps, etc.)
- Important phone numbers you will use
- How to get to another department
- How to hang a medication
- How to call the doctor
- What to do in the event of code or emergency (numbers involved)
- How to look at your work schedule
- How to request time off
- How to grab medications from the medication dispensing system
- Codes for locked rooms
- Where to find specific information in the patient's chart
- Who to call for medical equipment and supplies (environmental services, Biomed, Respiratory Therapy, central supply, etc.)

Off-Going Nurse Report

Your daily routine should be able to stand against the whirlwind. The whirlwind is the daily demands of Med-Surg nursing. Complexity is the enemy of execution, so you should make the layout of your daily routine as simple as possible.

The first two tasks in your daily routine will be:

1. Reviewing your patients' charts.
2. Gathering your patients' report from the off-going nurse at shift change.

Arrive to work as early as you are allowed to clock in. This will give you time to look over your patients' charts before you receive your patients' report from the off-going nurse. What is early? Ask your preceptor for the earliest time allowed for staff to clock in. You want to have a computer secured at this time. Remember, you will have to walk onto the unit and place your belongings in your break room, etc. You can't arrive "on time".

After clocking in, find where the charge nurse places the nurse assignments. Grab your patient assignments, then open your patients' charts to look over the essential parts. You should look over their orders, labs, and nurse's notes for any acute changes throughout the previous shift. Your preceptor will have to show you where the additional essential parts of your patient charts are found. (i.e. patient's vital signs, etc.)

Here are the essential parts of your patient's chart that I recommend you review:

MD orders | These are the active orders from the doctor for the nursing staff to follow.

Last MD note | The MD will identify your patient's problem list and all treatment for your patient's problem list and diagnoses.

Labs and imaging results | These will help you gather more information regarding your patient's current clinical picture.

Nurse's note | This may include information that couldn't otherwise be charted in the required daily charting. These are the highlights of your off-going nurse's shift.

Where should you write this information? Your nurse report sheet. The **MSRNPRO** report sheet was created to be a simple and efficient nurse report sheet. After you have written this information on your **MSRNPRO** report sheet, you can go meet the off-going nurse for your bedside report.

*(See Appendix A to view the **MSRNPRO** report sheet.)

Abbreviations

When gathering your morning reports, you can also abbreviate most common diagnoses. This will help you write your nurse report a little faster. Every little bit helps. These are only to be used for your report sheet and not for charting in your patient's electronic medical record.

- Hypertension (**HTN**)
- Congestive Heart Failure (**CHF**)
- Type II Diabetes Mellitus (**DMII**)
- Atrial Fibrillation (**Afib**)
- Acute Renal Failure (**ARF**)
- End-Stage Renal Disease (**ESRD**)
- Below Knee Amputation (**BKA**)
- Alcohol (**ETOH**)
- Chronic Obstructive Pulmonary Disease (**COPD**)
- Stroke (**CVA**)
- Pulmonary Embolism (**PE**)
- Deep Vein Thrombosis (**DVT**)
- Coronary Artery Bypass Graft (**CABG**)
- Headache (**HA**)
- Peptic ulcer Disease (**PUD**)
- Rheumatoid Arthritis (**RA**)
- Total Hip Replacement (**THR**)
- Total Knee Arthroplasty (**TKA**)
- Hyperlipidemia (**HLD**)

- Open Reduction Internal Fixation (**ORIF**)
- Acute Kidney Injury (**AKI**)
- Cancer (**CA**)

Bedside Report (Round 1)

Ask brilliant questions during shift change. The off-going nurse should know:

- Why the patient is still hospitalized
- If there will be any upcoming procedures for the patient
- The reason for any medications specific to inpatient treatment
- If there is a consultation for the patient to be seen by a specialty doctor

After writing down the information from the off-going nurse, go in the patient's room with the off-going nurse to be sure the patient looks the way the nurse described. This is Round 1. Rounding is basically checking on your patient with the intent to address any of their needs.

1. Introduce yourself to the patient. (Hi, my name is ______, I will be your nurse today.)
2. Update your patient's whiteboard with at least your name, the current date, and their doctor for the day.

3. Turn on the bed alarm if they are a high fall risk patient, assess your patient's IV site for redness, and check their IV fluid rate if IV fluid is infusing.
4. Advise the patient you are waiting for the doctors to round to gather more information on the goals for the day/night.
5. Ask if you can bring them anything when you come back with their medications. If you are a dayshift nurse, be sure they have ordered breakfast or know how to order breakfast. If they cannot order for themselves you should note that you will need to order their breakfast. Consider requesting an automatic tray for this patient if this is an option at your facility.

If a patient is NPO and awake in the morning during shift change, be sure to mention they are NPO and remove anything that they can eat or drink. Eating will delay their surgery or the procedure they have scheduled. Whoever ordered that procedure will be very upset about this and this mistake will prolong your patient's care.

After you have introduced yourself to all of your patients, you can sit down and finish writing in the missing information on your **MSRNPRO** report sheet. When this is complete, you will have a better idea of who is the sickest in your group. You will recognize who needs to be seen first, initiating the whole prioritization concept from nursing school.

When you go to give your medications, you should be **Thinking Forward** in hopes of putting out any potential fires. This is the time to bring your patient ice water, their food tray, their scheduled and prn medications, their new IV fluid bag, and whatever else they asked you to bring during Round 1. This is more than likely Round 2, the second time you've seen your patient for the day. Round 2 is part of every Med-Surg RN daily routine.

(Round 2)

If your patient needs help going to the bathroom, it's probably best to do it before you administer your medications. When you first get a patient up from bed, take into consideration the patient's level of mobility mentioned in your off-going nurse's report. Sometimes these assessments are inaccurate. If you have any doubt, ask for the help of your patient care tech or another nurse. Always use a gait belt when getting a patient up for the first time.

Medication Administration

Be prepared to be distracted when giving your medications. Look over each medication before you go into your patient's room, and always be sure that your vitals were checked before giving your medications. Your patient will start talking about random topics and may be requesting something outside of their due medications. Just remain focused on your task at hand. You should address their request before or after your medication administration. This is the best way to protect you and your patient. If taking the patient to the bathroom first will limit your distractions, do so.

You should always confirm all the "Rights of Medication Administration" for each medication you administer to your patients. Take your time, and review each medication and the dose with your patient before administering it. Be confident in the reason the patient is taking the medication.

If the patient does not know the reason they are taking an ordered medication or the medication does not line up with the patient's medical history, hold the medication and ask your preceptor or your charge nurse to help you **Figure It Out**. Calling around is an excellent method of **Figuring It Out.**

If I was attempting to figure this out, this is what I would do:

1. Consider the reason the patient was admitted. Also, consider their medical history for a reason the patient is taking the medication.
2. Search the hospital's medication database or the internet for the most common uses of the medication, then the uncommon uses.
3. Call the inpatient pharmacy and ask for their professional opinion.

4. Call the provider who ordered the medication if these other efforts were unsuccessful.

Head to Toe Assessment

Your daily routine includes your head-to-toe assessment. Your head-to-toe assessment should be a general one, but more focused on your patient's problem systems.

For example, a patient admitted for COPD exacerbation will receive a general head-to-toe assessment, but you will probably pay closer attention to this patient's respiratory findings versus comparing their legs for worsening signs of infection.

On the flip side, a patient admitted for bilateral lower extremity cellulitis will have his/her lungs auscultated because lung auscultation is a part of your standard quick head-to-toe assessment, but you will also evaluate their legs for signs of worsening infection. Both patients receive your general assessment in its normal flow, but there are areas that your assessments should become more focused. If you discover a new finding not mentioned in your nurse report, be sure to chart it in your flowsheet and notify the doctor if the finding warrants the doctor's attention.

Here's the normal flow of a quick head to toe assessment. Remember, you can refer to your clinical handbooks for the proper way to assess these systems. Ask your nurse preceptor to perform their usual assessment on one patient to give you a better point of reference. You should build and structure your assessments in a way that works best for you. You can add or remove any parts of this assessment that you feel are necessary for efficiency and essential to your patient care.

Neuro: Your introduction earlier in the morning partially assessed your patient's neuro/mental status. If your patient is a walking and talking adult, after holding a conversation with them, you will be able to tell if they are alert and oriented x 3-4. If you are concerned that you didn't adequately assess your patient's mental status, you can start your assessment by asking your patient about their night. Are they making sense? If they report any pain, consider this as you perform your physical assessment. Advise your patient that you will perform an assessment and then ask for their name and date of birth, comparing their answer to their identification band. Then, ask if they know the date and the reason they were admitted to the hospital.

Head: Scan their head for any abnormalities. We're talking about anything from wounds and lacerations to glasses or hearing aids.

Heart: Listen for abnormalities. Consider the patient's heart rate, murmurs, s1-s2, etc.

Lung: Glance at the clock to count their respirations per minute. You can usually count for 30 seconds and multiply your results times two for a regular rate, for irregular rates count for a full sixty seconds. Next, listen for abnormalities. Consider wheezing, crackles, rhonchi, etc.

Gastrointestinal (GI): Consider abnormal bowel sounds, absent/hyperactive bowel sounds, colostomy, etc. Ask the patient when they had their last bowel movement.

Genitourinary (GU): Ask if they are having any problems urinating. Do they have a foley catheter, suprapubic catheter urostomy, etc.? What are the characteristics of the urine?

Bilateral Upper Extremities: Scan skin for abnormalities and swelling. Make a note of skin temperature while assessing bilateral radial pulses and capillary refills.

Bilateral Lower Extremities: Scan skin for abnormalities and swelling. Make a note of skin temperature, while assessing bilateral dorsal pedal and posterior tibial pulses. Check capillary refills of all toes.

Lines: Assess all foreign lines going in or out of the patient for abnormalities. Confirm that any medication infusing into your patient's line is accurate and has an active order. Many times, medication rates are changed or discontinued during shift change. Check your MAR to confirm your infusion orders.

After you finish your assessment, be sure to exit your patient's room to chart your findings immediately.

Real-Time Charting

Chart as you go. This will prevent your charting from piling up. The number one reason nurses stay after their shift has ended is because they didn't chart in real-time. If you give your medication and then do your assessment in the mornings, after you step out of the patient's room, chart your assessment. Charting is important, but it isn't more important than your patient. Do not put off patient care to chart, but chart as soon as you break free from your patient's care. Do not provide patient care, then come out to socialize with others on the unit. Focus on your tasks, or it will cost you later.

Admissions

Med-Surg units are busy, and admissions will disrupt your routine. There will always be patients coming and going on a Med-Surg unit. Some will go for procedures, some discharging home, and some being admitted to your floor. Incoming patients are called "admissions." This is the process of a patient coming to your floor. The transferring department will call your floor and ask for you. Grab your **MSRNPRO** report sheet and fill it with all the information provided from the nurse of the transferring department. Most times you will be receiving an admission from the Emergency Department but it could be another unit or a procedural area like Radiology or the Operating Room.

Next, you will need to make sure all the supplies your patient will need are in the patient's room at their time of arrival. This is where **Thinking Forward** will prevent you from looking like a rookie. You should have a list of all the common things your patients will need when they come to your floor. If you don't have a list yet, refer to the list below:

- Update whiteboard
- Toothbrush
- Toothpaste*
- Bath soap*
- Lotion*
- Urinal (males)*
- Toilet hat (females)*
- Cup for water (Do not fill if your patient is NPO)
- Diet menu (Do not give if they are NPO)
- Non-slip socks*
- Blood pressure cuff*
- Sequential Compression Devices (SCD)
- SCD sleeves
- Hospital welcome packet*
- Primary IV tubing
- IV pump
- IV pole

- Telemetry leads/stickers
- Telemetry wires
- Towels*
- Extra hospital gown*

(*) items that every patient should receive

In a perfect world, all the applicable supplies should be neatly placed in the patient's room before their arrival. Don't forget that you can delegate this task to your patient care tech. Exercise your skill of **Thinking Forward**, consider having these supplies pre-stocked and bagged together on your unit for all new admissions.

After your patient arrives, you will complete an initial assessment on the patient and compare what you received in the report to the findings of your assessment. Be sure to check your patient's skin for signs of pressure injury, especially their buttocks, coccyx, and heels. If these wounds were present at the time of admission but not documented, your floor's nursing care will be to blame for the patient's skin breakdown.

After you have assessed your patient, you will ask your general admission questions and then give whatever medications are due at the time of the patient's arrival. Orient your patient to the floor and show them how to call for the nurse using the call light. Be sure they understand how to order food and use the television remote. These are small things that can trigger anxious patients when not proactively communicated. Do not stress yourself over admissions, you will get faster and faster at completing them.

The Most Underrated Nursing Skill

I don't hear this skill talked about nearly as much as it should be. If you have trouble with time management, one skill you can key in on is typing. I would recommend nurses make their goal to type at least 35 words per minute. The faster, the better. Increasing your typing speed will decrease your stress. This will save you so much time. Supremely clustering your patient care and quick typing is critical for efficient time management. However, these two are rarely mentioned when novice nurses explain their struggles with time management. Improve these two, and you will positively affect your time management.

Closing Out Your Shift

About three hours before the end of your shift, you should be **Thinking Forward** and preparing to close out your charting. Now is the time to update your **MSRNPRO** report sheet. When updating your **MSRNPRO** report sheet, here are a few areas to consider:

1. Procedures that were completed during your shift and the results.

2. Your patient's total intake and output for the shift.
3. Any acute changes.
4. Any PRN medications given during your shift.
5. Any unstable vital sign.
6. If you placed a nursing note for anything that isn't captured in your daily required nursing documentation.
7. Any behavioral concerns for the patient or their family member.
8. The plan for the next shift.

5 FIGHTING YOUR COMMUNICATION FEARS

"If your emotional abilities aren't in hand, if you don't have self-awareness, if you are not able to manage your distressing emotions, if you can't have empathy and have effective relationships, then no matter how smart you are, you are not going to get very far."

Daniel Goleman

Fear moves in when we overthink; usually when we're thinking of all the frightening possibilities that can occur at a particular place or time. Fear and anxiety will always be present in our work lives. However, you should approach your fears with prior preparation. The application of your learned knowledge will allow you to address your fears with a calmness that allows you to be your best analytical self. What if you don't have all the knowledge and skills needed to be a confident Med-Surg RN?

1. Start your preparation for those tasks in which you fear.
2. Be able to identify where the resources are that will calm your fears.

Prior preparation will help decrease your fear and anxiety about Medical-Surgical nursing. Below are topics that I believe cause the most anxiety on the typical Med-Surg nursing floor. You can exhale this very minute if you are committed to learning and applying this information. You will be prepared for those events that will more than likely catch your peers staring like a deer in headlights.

Difficult Conversations

Most of the time, the perceived threat of fear and our apprehensive thoughts are worse than having the actual conversation. As a Med-Surg RN PRO, you will be better prepared for the difficult conversations that are inevitable on a Med-Surg floor.

Learning how to communicate with difficult people will improve your work life, not theirs. Anxious and angry people must be given clear boundaries. Anger and anxiety can transfer quickly. You have to learn how to manage the escalation of emotions. As the Med-Surg RN PRO, you are the best person for the job. Create a mental vision of successful interactions with troublesome people. Your goal for difficult people should always be to maintain clear acceptable boundaries with a person who wouldn't otherwise be respectful of others in their moments of frustration. Make your vision more specific if you feel this will lead to better results. This especially applies to your patients and their family members. These two groups are where you will mostly find troublesome people.

You should never place yourself in harm's way because you are the nurse assigned to the patient. A person who is a jerk doesn't become a saint because they are a patient in a hospital. The hospital setting usually reveals who people are at their core. Do not argue with patients and do not put up with condescending comments or threats. As their nurse, you will be respectful, and they should be respectful as well. You are not someone's punching bag. If a patient is argumentative and aggressive, call security and ask them to come to speak with the patient. You can only provide your best care in an environment free from unnecessary emotional turmoil. This is your right as a professional. I have witnessed nurses argue with patients or chase patients down halls. Do not do this. If a patient wants to leave, let them leave. Chasing and begging patients is dangerous. Your hospital's security team should be adequately trained to de-escalate these types of patients. Call security and advise your charge nurse that you called security to help this patient set healthy boundaries. When security arrives, explain your requirements to care for this patient. If the patient agrees with the boundaries set, then you can continue caring for this person. If not, politely ask your charge nurse or house supervisor to find another caregiver. You should not make a habit of changing your patient assignments, but sometimes a seasoned nurse or a "no-nonsense" nurse will be a better fit for these patients. No nurse should be placed in harm's way for the sake of patient satisfaction. If this is the case, escalate your concerns to your leadership or HR until someone takes the matter seriously. Always document your interactions with the difficult patient using a timeline. When security is involved, they will also have documentation of their encounter with the person.

Always keep your tone and body language professional. Be yourself with difficult people. If you are upbeat, be upbeat. If you are the matter-of-fact type, be that, but do not let your compassion for your patient flee the scene because of their behaviors. Do not become angry or frustrated in a patient's room. This is where self-control is paramount. When you want to yell at the person, be silent or smile. If you can maintain this posture, you win. Self-assess your body language. Do not allow them to see your frustration with their behaviors. When they are becoming too much, it is okay to gracefully excuse yourself from their room. You may find a level of emotional relief after talking to a mature colleague about your stressful patient.

Remember: *The goal for managing a difficult person is to maintain clear acceptable boundaries for this person who wouldn't otherwise be respectful of others in their moments of frustration.*

Difficult People and Empathy

Some people are intimidating, domineering, and aggressive all in an effort to get their way in the hospital. There will be those who will complain to no end. These people blame others so that they will have the upper hand while they are in the nurse's care. Typically, their nurse will walk on eggshells when caring for them. They watch your every move and can't wait until their nurse makes a mistake. This is all part of caring for people.

Don't attempt to change a difficult person. Do not take their comments and behavior personally. Their behavior has more to do with underlying emotional issues than anything you may have done specifically. There's a possibility that you can neutralize a person's frustration using empathy. Empathy can sometimes de-escalate explosive situations.

Never agree with their behaviors but acknowledge their feelings in the moment and respond with these five phrases:

1. "So, you feel that..."

You should hear them out and clarify their concerns.

2. "I can see why you're upset."

Empathy creates an environment of care and concern, not confrontation.

3. "I am sorry that I didn't meet your expectations on this occasion."

Show your acknowledgment of their wishes.

4. "What can I do to make this better for you?"

Respond with asking for their input on a solution.

5. "Thank You for bringing this to my attention. I will work on a solution!"

Keep the person updated on the solution. Be clear on what you can or cannot do.

After the out-of-control person is calmer, you can set healthy boundaries for your future communications. Use fewer words in your communication with difficult people. Mastering the above phrases can be crucial to maintaining your sanity. Less conversation is often more effective with difficult people.

Unfriendly Coworkers

I've noticed one type of person who consistently breaks through social barriers in the workplace. It is usually the person with the right attitude towards their work and their colleagues. Having the right attitude will have a huge impact on your work relationships. Your thoughts will constantly influence your attitude. Take honest inventory of your thoughts. How you feel about yourself and how you feel about others will determine your attitude. What we believe about ourselves impacts our ability to connect with others. If you consistently have negative thoughts about yourself, then you will think others consistently have negative thoughts about you as well. You should see yourself through a realistic and positive lens and assume others view you this way too. Even when others don't see you this way, remember that a negative person's opinion is pretty worthless in our line of work. The right attitude towards unfriendly coworkers will lift you above the rest of your team. This increases your value on your floor. I've never met a nurse who doesn't want to work with someone who has a great attitude.

However, you can't allow unfriendly coworkers or difficult people to emotionally abuse you. The same boundaries we talked about earlier regarding your patients and their families apply to your coworkers as well. Set firm boundaries regarding the level of respect you expect while working with your coworker.

If necessary, consider using the five phrases of empathy listed above to maintain your relationship with an unfriendly coworker. Sincerely listen to the person's request. If this person frequently has unreasonable requests of you, voice your concerns to the person. If the issue is impacting the quality of your work life or patient care, minimize your communication with this person until you two can further resolve the matter with your nurse supervisor or nurse manager.

Delegation Phrases

These are phrases you can use every day to decrease your communication fears while delegating tasks on your Med-Surg unit.

"Would you be so kind as to..."

"Would you take a few seconds to..."

"Are you available to ... for me?"

"Do you mind grabbing... for me?"

If the person says "Yes" they will complete your request, always say "Thank You!" Even if you don't like their tone and attitude. Be consistent with your own attitude and responses. If their body language or demeanor is rude enough to be addressed, do so after the task is completed. It's usually a good idea to address communication issues that arise on the unit sooner rather than later.

Communicating with Physicians

If there is a clinical need that requires calling a MD, grab a set of vital signs before placing the call.

Be sure that there has been a recent set of vitals completed on the patient. Recent meaning within the last 5-15 minutes at least. While waiting for a call back from the MD, do not start any task that you can't easily stop.

You should have the patient's chart open and expect questions from the MD that are specific to your reason for calling. Why? Because you are on your way to becoming a Med-Surg RN PRO, and you are always **Thinking Forward**. The MD will likely ask you something that can easily be found in the patient's chart. (i.e., questions about medications, lab values, the patient's health history, their medication allergies, recent vital signs, etc.) Also, have your pen and paper ready to write new orders.

Use the SBAR below as a guide when speaking with Physicians

Situation: This is (nurse's name) the nurse for the patient (first and last name) in room number ___ on the hospital's ___ floor.

Background: The patient was admitted for ____ but I'm calling because of (reason for call).

Assessment: Report whatever clinical findings are new and relevant. If nothing, skip to the Recommendation.

Recommendation: Ask for the order you think will address the issue or ask for the MD's recommendation for the event. If the doctor gives you a verbal order over the phone, always read back the order.

Practicing is the best way to prepare, this preparation can eliminate your fear.

Here's an exercise for you...

Watch your preceptor as they reach out to a MD. Take notes on what he/she's doing, and later ask if you can call or page the MD when the opportunity arises again. Ask your preceptor to assist and correct you during and after your call or page. If it's over the phone, see if your preceptor can listen to your conversation in a three-way set up. This provides your preceptor an opportunity to add any information they think may help you better communicate with the doctor.

6 FIGHTING YOUR CLINICAL FEARS

"Inaction breeds doubt and fear. Action breeds confidence and courage. If you want to conquer fear, do not sit home and think about it. Go out and get busy."

Dale Carnegie

Most nurses are worried about the worst-case scenario when it comes to their patients. This worry can be reduced when a nurse knows how to identify such a scenario. If you know what a sick patient looks like, you should be just fine.

This section includes the most common conditions you will see in a patient who is getting sick. After receiving your report from the off-going RN, briefly start **Thinking Forward** to the worst-case scenario for each of your patients based on their admitting diagnosis and present clinical findings. General knowledge about these conditions should provide a solid foundation for you to confidently identify changes within your assigned patients. I will not review all the details of these conditions. I assume you are aware of each since you've graduated and passed the NCLEX. This is where you will apply your critical thinking knowledge from nursing school. You may hear about patients getting "sick." This means they are clinically getting worse. As a Med-Surg RN PRO, you will be able to identify changes in your patients. This section is not comprehensive and was intentionally created using simple terms. Sometimes less is more. Review this section frequently to combat the fear of these events.

In all of these events, immediately contact your charge nurse and state these words, "Hey (charge nurse's name), please come look at my patient. I think they are getting sicker."

All changes in your patient's condition should immediately be followed by checking a full set of your patient's vital signs.

Sepsis

Sepsis can occur with the majority of the Med-Surg patient population. Learn to zero in on these things to consider if your patient is becoming septic.

Short Term Interventions:

- Ask the charge nurse or a seasoned nurse you trust to look at your patient and ask for their thoughts on your patient's condition.

- Notify the provider of the changes. **Thinking Forward**, you should expect to receive a few new orders.
- After receiving new orders, this patient is your highest priority for the next hour. This really applies to any patient who is getting "sick", despite the reason for their clinical decline.
- Ask your charge nurse or a buddy to check on your other patients while you address this patient.

Questions to Ask Yourself:

- Is the temperature higher or lower than normal?
- Is there a possible infection?
- Has there been a change in mental status (confused or drowsy)?
- Does the patient have a new complaint of severe pain or not feeling well?

Things to Review:

- Check your patient's vital signs immediately. Compare these findings to the patient's previous vital signs or results.
- Fever (>100.4 F), chills, sweats, change in mentation/confusion, lethargy, hypotension (systolic BP<90), tachycardia (HR >100), tachypnea (RR>20), oxygen saturation < 94%, reduced urine

output, elevated lactic acid, positive blood or wound cultures, etc.

- New orders placed by the physician after your notification of the event.

Bleeders

Patients who have a history of gastrointestinal bleeding, recent surgery, receiving coagulation therapy, or bleeding disorders that suddenly have an elevated heart rate, low blood pressure, paleness, and lethargy may have internal bleeding. These signs and symptoms may also be found in the hypovolemic patient.

Short Term Interventions:

- Ask the charge nurse or a seasoned nurse you trust to look at your patient and ask for their thoughts on your patient's condition.
- Grab a full set of vitals.
- Check those vitals every five minutes or whatever your hospital policy says.
- Notify the provider of the changes. **Thinking Forward,** you should expect to receive a few new orders.

Question to Ask Yourself:

- Are there any external areas where you can spot the patient from bleeding (surgical sites, wounds, rectum, drain sites, etc.)?

- Where can you find a pressure bag to administer a bolus if ordered?
- Does the patient have a working IV to administer any fluid bolus or blood transfusion?
- Who can draw STAT labs if you can't? Specifically, a complete blood count (CBC).

Things to Review:

- Assess the patient's vitals for a negative trend in the patient's blood pressure.
- New orders placed by the physician after your notification of the event.

Respiratory Distress

Patients experiencing respiratory distress are usually easy to notice. The patient will tell you or your general nursing knowledge will alert you.

Short Term Interventions:

- Ask the charge nurse or a seasoned nurse you trust to look at your patient and ask for their thoughts on your patient's condition
- Grab a full set of vitals, paying close attention to their respiratory rate and oxygen saturation. If it's less than 92%, grab a nasal cannula and place the patient on oxygen starting at two Liters per minute. Increase the rate as needed to bring the pa-

tient above 94%. Do not exceed six liters per minute unless otherwise ordered. (Do this only if your hospital policy permits RN to place patients in respiratory distress on oxygen.)

- Call and ask the respiratory therapist assigned to your patient to come and look at the patient for you. They are a great resource and the respiratory system expert.
- Notify the provider of the changes. **Thinking Forward**, you should expect to receive a few new orders.

For patients who are breathing rapidly (>25 breaths per minute) accompanied by a decrease in their oxygen saturation despite the above intervention, consider calling your hospital's Rapid Response Team or Rapid Assessment Team (RRT/RAT).

Also, consider calling your hospital's Rapid Response Team or Rapid Assessment Team for patients who are breathing slowly (<6 breaths per minute). You will need to provide rescue breaths with a bag-valve mask. The bag-valve mask is found on your floor's crash cart. Give one breath every six seconds. Be sure your patient continues to have a pulse. Check for a pulse every two minutes until you have the RRT/RAT team in the room to help.

Questions to Ask Yourself:

- Did you recently give the patient any narcotics?
- Does this patient have a history of anxiety?
- Does this patient have a history of respiratory failure, heart failure, or any chronic respiratory disease?
- Is this patient receiving intravenous fluids with a history of heart failure?

Things to Review:

- Ask your patient to breathe deeply if they can follow commands.
- Is your charge nurse, RRT/RAT team, and MD at the bedside?
- Look over medications and think through the medications that may have caused respiratory distress.
- If the patient's respiratory distress is caused by medications, consider getting an order to give Narcan (naloxone) to reverse the symptoms of medication overdose.

Stroke

If you walk into your patient room and their mentation has changed, but they have no history of infection, you may be witnessing an active stroke. You will need to use the F.A.S.T. assessment for this event.

Short term interventions: Ask your patient to complete these commands to complete your F.A.S.T. stroke assessment.

- Face | **Ask your patient to smile**. Does one side of their face droop?
- Arms | **Ask your patient to raise both arms**. Does one side appear weaker than the other?
- Speech | **Ask your patient to repeat a simple phrase like, "I can't wait to go home to rest in my bed."** Does their speech sound slurred?
- Time | **Review your memory and patient records for symptom onset or last known normal.** When was the last time someone saw this patient, and they were acting normal? If your patient is having a stroke, time is brain.

*You can review their coagulation labs if they have been completed. aPTT, PT/INR, Heparin Anti-Xa, platelets, etc.

- Grab a full set of vitals. Notify the provider of the changes. **Thinking Forward**, you should expect to receive a few new orders.

Be prepared to receive STAT orders for CT Head or MRI of the brain. You will more than likely need to push your patient's bed down to the procedural department. Ask someone (charge or seasoned nurse) to go with you to the procedural department. It's very common for two nurses to go down with the patient during these types of events. The other nurse should be Advanced Cardiovascular Life Support (ACLS) certified. Provide oxygen if the patient is hypoxemic.

Questions to Ask Yourself:

- Does this patient have a history of stroke, hypertension, blood clots, atrial fibrillation, smoking, high cholesterol, diabetes, etc.?
- Where will your patient transfer to if they are having a stroke?
- Is this patient on telemetry monitoring? Afib?

Things to Review:

- Check your patient's vital signs immediately. While checking your patient's vital signs, you should assess the patient's mental status.
- Can the patient confirm their name, date of birth, where they are, and the date?
- New orders placed by the physician after your notification of the event.

Hypoglycemia (Low Blood Sugar)

Stroke and low blood sugar symptoms look very similar. If your patient's mentation changes and they are using blood glucose altering medications, they may be hypoglycemic.

Short Term Interventions:

- Grab a full set of vital signs and check the patient's blood sugar.
- If your patient's blood sugar is low, follow your facility's hypoglycemia protocol.
- If your hospital does not have a hypoglycemia protocol, and the patient can follow commands, give the patient two orange juices to drink and crackers to eat.
- If your patient cannot follow commands, you need to request an order for Dextrose (D50) IV push or Glucagon IM.
- Recheck their blood glucose after you treat it. Continue to treat per your hospital's hypoglycemia protocol.

Questions to Ask Yourself:

- Does this patient pass the F.A.S.T. assessment but have a history of diabetes?
- Is the patient taking a blood glucose altering medication (Insulin, Glucophage, etc.)?
- What was their last capillary blood glucose number?
- Does the patient have a working PIV?

Things to Review:

- Have you recently given any insulin?

- Do you have an order to check the patient's blood glucose?
- Do you have an order for PRN Dextrose? If not, notify MD and request any orders you need.
- Speaking with the charge nurse regarding orders that the patient may need specific to this event.

Cardiac Arrest

If you walk into your patient's room and they are unresponsive and not breathing normally, this may be a cardiac arrest situation.

Short Term Interventions:

If your patient is full code, you will immediately carry out your Adult Basic Life Support (CPR) training. Stay calm and complete the following 3 steps.

1. Calmly ask the patient if he/she is okay. If no response, check for a carotid pulse for 5-10 seconds.
2. If there is no pulse, calmly press the code blue button.
3. Flatten the bed and start CPR chest compressions.

Continue CPR until told otherwise by the code blue emergency team. When someone arrives with the crash cart, remember to place the backboard under the patient to give effective compressions. Someone will place the AED pads on the patient while you are performing compressions. Someone should get in place to provide rescue breaths, as well.

The crash cart and code team will arrive, and there will be someone who is ACLS certified who will probably take over the code. Your responsibility is to initiate Adult Basic Life Support (BLS). Your goal is to get your patient's blood flowing to the vital organs as soon as you recognize your patient does not have a pulse. This is your goal until the code team arrives. Even after someone replaces you from doing compressions, make yourself available to answer questions about the patient's history or the events that led up to the code. You can look at your report sheet to answer the questions during this time. The perfect situation would include looking through the patient's electronic chart via a computer to answer their questions.

Remember to always stay in the room if your patient is in trouble. Don't leave unless someone asks you to run and grab something. Make sure your patient has a working PIV. If you think the PIV isn't dependable, ask someone to place another one for you.

No matter the outcome of this emergency, your charge nurse should be able to assist you in all the next steps.

Questions to Ask Yourself:

- Has anyone connected the AED pads to your patient?

- Does this patient have a working PIV?
- Has RT arrived to provide rescue breaths with a bag valve mask?
- Does the oxygen on the wall work?
- Has anyone set up wall suction?
- Have any new orders been placed since the event?

Things to Review:

- As the bedside nurse, stay in the patient's room until the emergency team leader has finished asking you questions about your patient's history.
- As a newer nurse you are more than capable of performing CPR with the other providers. Volunteering to do so is a good idea. Experience is the best teacher for events like these.
- Your goal rate for compressions is 100 - 120 per minute at a depth 2 - 2.5 inches. You should perform 30 compressions and then 2 rescue breaths. Verbalize exactly when you want another provider to replace you in giving compressions. This is usually after you finish your set of 30 compressions. (i.e "Please replace me after this set of 30 is complete.")
- Common key roles during a code: medication nurse, scribe, code leader, CPR providers (who rotate to prevent exhaustion), respiratory therapist, anesthesia, charge nurse, chaplain, bedside nurse, and security. **Thinking Forward**, now is a

good time to make yourself familiar with the responsibilities of each of these roles.

- What does your charge nurse recommend you do while the code is continuing or when it's finished?
- When the emergency is over, be sure to look over the drawers in the crash cart with the permission of your charge nurse. This is a good time to become familiar with your unit's crash cart.
- If family is present the chaplain can comfort this person. If you are upset about this event, be sure to speak to your chaplain regarding your feelings, as well.

It's always a superb idea to review your American Heart Association Adult Basic Life Support (CPR) steps frequently (weekly) at the start of your Med-Surg experience. When no one else is prepared, the Med-Surg RN PRO is prepared and **Thinking Forward** regarding the event of a cardiac arrest.

YOUR FIRST SEVEN SHIFTS

7

"Constant attention by a good nurse may be just as important as a major operation by a surgeon."

Dag Hammarskjold

Your internship/residency/orientation should have individual goals for each shift. These goals will need to be checked off by your preceptor, Nurse Manager, and Nurse Educator. Each shift, I have a few additional goals for you to apply if you want to make the most of your Med-Surg learning program. The objectives given by your hospital are your primary concern. I have included a few goals that will complement your program. These will not hinder your overall floor learning experience. Honestly, I believe it will add more value to your Med-Surg nursing foundation. These are the subjects I wished would have been added to my program.

The Day Before Shift 1

You should be pumped. Why? You get to size up your next challenge. You are preparing to go to your unit to assess the best method to defeat a five to six patient assignment. The day before is mostly mental preparation and organization. You are entering the world of nursing where the possibilities are endless. Shift by shift, you will defeat this first year to gain access to the exceptional stability of the nursing profession. You can and will do it. Preparation is key for your first shift.

Take a deep breath because tomorrow you are mostly covering the basics. You have no reason to be anxious. However, I will say that you should be prepared.

Here's a list of supplies I recommend:

- Stethoscope
- MSRNPRO report sheet
- Dependable Watch
- Comfortable shoes (Asics, Brooks, Hoka, etc.)
- Comfortable scrubs
- Badge
- Pens
- Permanent marker
- Clinical Skills Handbook
- Snacks and lunch or payment for lunch
- Your daily medications (if necessary)
- Water bottle
- Backpack or shoulder bag
- A notepad or index cards for note-taking

Shift 1

It's showtime! You will not be asked to do much on this day, but I strongly recommend that you try to accomplish these three goals:

1. Develop a consistent habit of notetaking. You will learn a bunch of information on this day. You cannot record all the information you learn, but you should write all the information you think will be important to know. How do you determine which information is important to write? If you aren't sure, you should ask your preceptor, "If you were me, would you write this down?" Write the learned information in your designated note-taking area. Don't panic if you fail to take note of a routine task, as you will very likely have another opportunity to do so.
2. Learn how to find information about your patients that will allow you to fill in your MSRN-PRO report sheet.
3. Find simple examples throughout your day in which you can use **Thinking Forward** and **Figuring It Out**. Remember, **Thinking Forward** is knowing or considering what your next task will be. **Figuring It Out** is your ability to successfully conquer the challenges before you by utilizing all of your available and thinkable resources. These two will turn you into a problem-solving ma-

chine. Talk through your considerations with your preceptor.

Early in your shift, ask your preceptor to delegate one simple task to you, and write this task down. This should be something easy that you can do without a doubt. Complete the task and cross it off your list. Later in the shift, ask for three more simple tasks, write them down, then cross them off of your list. A little later, ask for five more tasks, write them down, and cross them off. Your focus at this point isn't the tasks themselves. I want you to get in the habit of writing down your tasks, gathering your supplies, and completing the tasks. As your days' progress, you will continue to write, gather, and complete.

Below are few topics you can consider during Shift 1

- Was there anything you liked about your preceptor's daily routine or patient care strategy?
- Remember, there should always be an area on your report sheet to write tasks.
- Identify an area where you will take notes.
- Don't be afraid to ask to complete tasks for your preceptor's most stable patient.

Shift 2

I expect you to be more hands-on this shift compared to the last shift. Here are your three goals for this shift:

1. Continue to take great notes and search for opportunities to **Think Forward** and **Figure It Out** during this shift.
2. Use your bedside nurse report and your patient's electronic chart to completely fill in your **MSRN-PRO** report sheet.
3. Complete a quick head-to-toe assessment on as many of your preceptor's patients as time will allow.

Shift 3

You have probably learned more than you imagined you could learn in your last 48 hours on the floor. You are well on your way to becoming a Med-Surg RN PRO! Here are three goals for this shift:

1. Use **Thinking Forward** and **Figuring It Out** to complete "Round 1" and "Round 2" for at least one of your assigned patients. If you want to gain more practice, do this for more than one of your assigned patients.
2. Start your running list of numbers for other departments. Ask your preceptor for the phone numbers to the most frequently called departments and floors. This list can be written in the

same notepad that you are taking notes in. (Hint: ask for your facility's phone operator number.) Remember, you can use your facility's phone operator to find any phone number.

3. Watch and take notes while your preceptor gathers their report during shift change. At the end of the shift, ask if you can give the nurse report to the incoming nurse for one of your patients using your **MSRNPRO** report sheet.

Shift 4

Thinking Forward and **Figuring It Out** should be part of your initial mental processing whenever you have a question to answer from your preceptor. Here are three goals for this shift:

1. Gather report for all of your assigned patients as if your preceptor is present. Ask brilliant questions. It is usually best to ask questions when the off-going nurse is finished giving a report, politely interject if you think you may forget your question before they are finished with their report.
2. Know what a sick patient looks like. If you can identify this early on, you will know it when you are nursing without a preceptor. Identify the sickest patient in your preceptor's assignment. Go check him or her out. Get the visual. Tell your preceptor, "I want to always know what a sick patient looks like so I can best prioritize my care."

3. Complete "Round 2" for 2 of your patients but be more prepared than you were in shift 3 by utilizing **Thinking Forward**. Will your patient need fresh ice and water, fresh non-slip socks, supplies to take a shower independently, a linen change, as needed pain or nausea medication, insulin from a locked location, a new bag of continuous fluid or replacement of electrolytes per electrolyte sliding scale?

Shift 5

You have a general idea of where some things are on your floor. Sometimes the one irritating issue is trying to find something you need when you need it. Here are three goals for this shift:

1. Start working on completing the "List of things the MSRNPRO knows."
2. Continue to update your list of all your important numbers throughout this shift.
3. Ask for a walking tour to CT, MRI, ED, GI LAB, ICUs, Cath LAB, and other departments that may require the primary nurse to take an unstable patient. Write down the routes in your note section if this helps you recall where these locations are. Why? You will rarely need to walk to these departments and likely forget where they are.

*(See Appendix B for the List of Things the MSRNPRO Knows.)

Shift 6

Technology and nursing are closely related. Here are three goals for this shift:

1. Immediately after you complete "Round 2," chart your assessment for that patient.
2. Find out your typing speed. If it is less than 35 words per minute, commit to working on your typing speed outside of work. There are free typing exercises on websites like www.typingclub.com.
3. Recall where to find your patient information in your patient electronic chart without help from your preceptor.

Bonus Goals

Your first six shifts covered a few foundational skills that will allow you to be less stressed and more proactive in your journey of becoming a Med-Surg RN PRO. Here are three more goals to wrap up your first two weeks.

1. Start your next shift, recognizing that you are committed to **Task Management**. Remember, **Task Management** is safely concentrating on a single task while considering the steps of the next

in a way that prepares you to effectively complete an immediate or larger task.

2. Identify three tasks that you will use your **Thinking Forward** and **Figuring It Out** skills to complete the **Task Management** of a larger task during your shift.
3. Complete all necessary communication between doctor and nurse for your assigned patients. Allow your preceptor to assist but be sure you are the one reaching out to the doctors throughout your shift.

SIMPLIFYING WEEKS 3 - 8

8

"You are capable of more than you know. Choose a goal that seems right for you and strive to be the best, however hard the path. Aim high. Behave honorably. Prepare to be alone at times, and to endure failure. Persist! The world needs all you can give."

E. O. Wilson

Week 3

Computer charting is a lifesaver for the nurse administering medications. Many hospitals have a charting and scanning process in place that saves us so much time. However, there is always room for improvement. This week, you should become more efficient at safely administering your medications. The keyword here is "safely." Never rush to administer medications. Think about two habits in your medication administration routine that you can improve on. Work to improve those two habits this week and never look back at your old habits again. Use

Figuring It Out to produce the outcome you desire. Here are two examples:

1. Forgetting to reassess your patient's pain level after administering an as needed pain medication. (Set a timer on your phone and return to your patient's room after the timer alarms to see if the pain medication relieved your patient's pain.) In this example, you are **Figuring It Out** by using your phone timer as a resource.
2. Taking too long to administer your medications because your patient is very talkative and distracting. (Set a time limit for your medication administration and stick to your guns. 10-15 minutes should be long enough in most cases. This is a struggle that all newer nurse's experience. You should have an exit strategy and phrase that you will use to break free after your task is finished. Ask your preceptor or a colleague to check in with you when your time is up. In this example, you are **Figuring It Out** by utilizing your preceptor or colleague as a resource for being time efficient.)

Thinking Forward, are there any medications that can be moved to an earlier or later time to cluster your care? Ask your preceptor how to move medications that are not time sensitive. (i.e. multivitamins, allergy medications, proton pump inhibitors, etc.) You're clustering your care knowing you can better use your free time providing patient care, taking your break, or completing incomplete charting instead of bringing your patient these medications multiple times throughout your shift.

If there are any medications you are unfamiliar with, review and research these medications before you step foot in your patient's room. In doing this, you are continuing to **Think Forward** by reviewing all medications so you will have a proper understanding of the medications before administering them to your patient. **Thinking Forward** is beneficial in this case because you are considering the fact that your patient may not be familiar with the medication and may ask you the reason he or she is being given the medication. You'll be prepared for these questions.

Week 4

Remember, every nurse has a unique way of providing care. This week, consider the best way to perform your quick head-to-toe assessment. Can you identify one thing that slows you down with all of your head-to-toe assessments? This is one area you need to address. Set small measurable goals for yourself. In your considerations, realize that consistency is vital. Here are a few parts of your assessment to consider becoming more consistent and efficient with:

- ***The way you want your assessment to flow.*** Are you assessing the areas of focus first or after you complete your general head to toe assessment?
- ***Ideally, how long should the average assessment take?*** This is very important in your daily time management.
- ***Do you want to complete your dressing changes per the MD's order during your head-to-toe assessment or later in the day?***
- ***Should you make a priority of completing your head-to-toe assessment before you meet your patient's request to get out of the bed for the first time in your shift?***
- ***Do you need to flush any drains or tubes?*** This is an excellent time to do so, as well as record the output in urinals, drains, etc. If so, where in the process would you prefer to do so, at the end of your assessment or before beginning your assessment.

Use **Figuring It Out** to successfully conquer the challenges of your quick head-to-toe assessment by utilizing all of your available and thinkable resources. Consider what your preceptor can do to help you successfully meet your intended goals.

Thinking Forward, you should have a quiet place in mind that you can chart the findings of your assessment immediately after you finish your assessment. This is the best way to chart an accurate assessment. You are **Thinking Forward** by identifying your next step after physically performing your assessment. Putting it off is one thing that many nurses make an awful habit of, but trust me when I say that it leads to many headaches. The perfect scenario would include having a computer in the room and charting your assessment in the patient's room. This is very possible for confused patients and those patients who don't mind you hanging out in their room. Most of your patients will distract you with multiple requests or make it downright uncomfortable for you to hang out in their room while charting. In most instances, it's best to leave your patient's room after you complete your head-to-toe assessment.

Week 5

Charting, the struggle is real! I recommend dedicating more than one week of focused time to being intentional about charting at the actual time a task is performed. This method of charting is called charting in "real-time". Especially when you are performing your "Round 2" for your assigned patients. Chart all you can immediately after or during these rounds. Especially your head-to-toe assessment. Ask your preceptor and other nurses for ways that will help you chart quicker. Try to apply at least one shortcut to your routine from each nurse you ask. Write these shortcuts down, and continue to use them if they are beneficial to you.

Also, we can't forget how closely related our typing speed is to our overall charting time. This week is an excellent time to continue working on your typing speed. Are you typing at least 35 words per minute? Use **Figuring It Out** to identify your best method for charting in real-time. Your most valuable resources will be the people on your unit who seem to sit around talking. They have found something that works. I'm recommending incorporating their methods with this exception: do not adopt any bad habits. If it doesn't sound right, then it probably isn't. If they are recommending you take a "shortcut" that requires you to compromise your work, do not take their advice. Find someone who is completing their charting in a reasonable amount of time and maintaining a high level of integrity. Faster is only better when you are consistently, safely, and efficiently completing all the tasks that are expected of you by your leadership.

You could more than likely figure out which real-time charting methods work best on your own, but this can take many shifts. I'd rather you become a Med-Surg RN PRO quicker through the wisdom and experience of others. I can promise you that you will get faster and faster the more you intentionally try to become better. Please don't think that all the quicker nurses have a secret formula for charting. They should be able to help you identify a few tricks they've learned through their charting experiences, but another factor in the quick completion of their charting is the repetitive pattern that they've had for many shifts. You, too, will experience this one day.

Unfortunately, you will not be able to chart in real-time on many occasions. In this event, use your **Thinking Forward** skills to create a plan to find a computer and chart what you need to chart as soon as you are free to do so. (Hint: Your plan might include you writing a list of your abnormal assessment findings until you can get to the nearest computer.)

Week 6

This is the week you should use **Figuring It Out** to complete the "List of things the MSRNPRO knows." Knowing these things will lay a great foundation for your list of resources. This knowledge will be key as you continue your nursing career. Use your **Thinking Forward** skills to add any other items you think are essential for you to know on your floor.

Two things you can add to your list are:

1. The various ways to call a "Code Blue." (Calling through an operator, pressing the code blue button, etc.)
2. The quickest method for calling your hospital's "Rapid Response Team" or Rapid Assessment Team" to your unit if your patient is clinically declining.

Week 7

What if you page a doctor, and you do not get a response?

This week, use your **Figuring It Out** skill to answer this question. Write down your findings. This will eventually happen, and you don't want to be in the middle of a crisis asking your preceptor or another nurse this question. Knowing what to do before it's time to do it reduces the stress of a stressful event.

Have you run into any trouble with communicating with providers? Were there any communication misunderstandings, large or small? You should use this week to improve your method of communicating with all providers. You are **Thinking Forward** because when this challenge arises, you will be prepared to move to the next step in getting in contact with your difficult to reach provider.

Find out if you have providers who have a reputation of requiring a method of communication that differs from the normal process of communicating with in-house providers.

Week 8

Now that you've been on your floor for a few weeks, use this week to find a mentor. Your preceptor is the bomb, but you want someone you can voice your concerns to and then receive trusted advice from. Someone you aspire to be like as an RN. Meaningful work and meaningful relationships matter. In my experience, encouragement from those who we respect is powerful. This is the person who will consistently encourage and possibly correct you. There will be times when a patient or staff member makes a comment that discourages you. I'm helping you in your **Thinking Forward** by setting you up to have a person you can talk to on the hard days. Never let a patient or staff member validate your worth. They will have the power to deny your worth if so. The fact that you have the desire to read this book shows that you are more than capable and have a promising future just around the corner.

Create a plan in which you will check in with your mentor. This can be a formal meeting or an informal check in with each other via text. If you are having trouble finding an excellent mentor, ask your unit's nurse manager for his or her recommendation. Your unit manager is a great resource in **Figuring It Out**. The goal is to complete this task by the end of the week, but do not rush this task.

Also, use this week to organize all of your notes and lists of resources. You are **Thinking Forward** to the day that you will be on your own. These notes will be your best friend as you continue to sharpen your **Figuring It Out** skills. Remove all the items you are confident in finding. Create a shortlist of those things that you still need to refer to your list to find. Find time to update (adding and subtracting) items throughout your first year on the floor.

MANAGING MONTHS 3-8

9

"Our goals can only be reached through a vehicle of a plan, in which we must fervently believe, and upon which we must vigorously act. There is no other route to success."

Pablo Picasso

Month 3

March through these next two months using your previous shift experiences to identify areas that need more intentional time for strengthening. You have been on your floor long enough to recognize that you have learned so much, but you still have so much more to learn.

At first glance, the information in this book, combined with your progression through your nurse orientation, may seem like a lot of information. You are right but remember, this is recent information that you will continue to build on. You want to be intentional about plugging in the content of Med-Surg RN PRO into the holes of your daily routine to create a better Med-Surg experience for you and your patients.

To do this, you have to complete all the goals we have covered up to this point in a satisfactory manner. This is a wonderful time to use your **Figuring It Out** skill to identify any goals that were partially completed or entirely completed but could be improved. **Thinking Forward,** you understand that continuous improvement is a staple of healthcare and is dear to nursing professionals that create the compassionate fabric of our healthcare system.

Months 4-6 - PRO-TIPS

If you aren't already, you will soon be off orientation and on your own. This is the perfect time to introduce you to the wonderful world of PRO-Tips. You can review your PRO-Tips at any point after orientation. PRO-Tips are the knowledge and wisdom that will separate you from those with the same level of professional nursing experience. You are about to read them, but I want to encourage you to remember and apply the PRO-Tips when you are independently working your unit in the months to come.

Put Out Those Fires

Patients will usually call at the most inopportune time. To help with this, round frequently and complete their requests so that they don't pile up. Round every 1-2 hours. Take a brief walk around the unit to check on your patients. Put out your fires early by rounding. Patients admitted with chest pain may need pain medication. Patients with a urinary tract infection may need help to use the bathroom because of urinary frequency. Patients admitted for nausea may need their prn nausea medication. Think of the things your patient may need as you round (i.e. freshwater, toothbrush, toothpaste, bath soap, and towels for a shower, urine emptied from urinals, drains emptied, pain medication, etc.).

Raise the Bed

Always raise your patient's bed when caring for your patient. Do not get into the habit of bending over to push or pull a patient. If you do, it is only a matter of time before you hurt your back. You only get one back, take excellent care of it.

Preceptor Options

Be sure you have a preceptor you can be honest with and learn from. If you and your preceptor do not mesh well after two or three months, ask your nurse manager for other preceptor options.

Be Cool as a Cucumber

Always resolve conflict as soon as possible while remaining mature. With this being said, it is perfectly acceptable to walk away to cool off if needed.

Don't Over Commit

It's always best to under-promise and over-deliver. This can apply to any task you are promising to complete for your patient. We can use prn medications as an example. Do not promise a patient you will bring their medication at an exact time. When you cannot do so, it will disappoint them. So, saying you will bring the medication within a 10–15-minute window of the time that the medication is due should be sufficient. Never say that you'll be right back, or that you'll be back in a minute. You can say, "I'll get back here as soon as I can" or "My goal is to have the medication here for you in the next 20 minutes. Remember, the patient is part of the care team, so it is appropriate to ask them to press the nurse button to remind you just in case a distraction takes you away from your goal.

Change Your Gloves

If you are working in a room for a while, look for reasons to change gloves. If you pick up something off the floor and subsequently need to touch your patient, change gloves. If you have to give medication and then dump a urinal, change gloves. Change gloves after you've touched anything associated with bodily fluids when you have to continue working in your patient's room. This isn't to be wasteful but to be mindful when you may otherwise be so focused that you overlook unsanitary patient care practice.

No Doubt...This Will Humble You

There's one thing I can guarantee that has humbled every nurse who has ever stepped foot on a Med-Surg floor for a year or two. This one thing is the roller clamp to your IVPB. As a novice nurse, it is a good habit to check the chamber of all of your fluids before you leave the room. If you do this, maybe you can be the first nurse ever to never come back later, only to realize your patient never received their medications because you didn't unclamp their secondary line. This always happens when you least expect it, and it will definitely humble and embarrass you. The average novice nurse doesn't know to be on high alert after hanging an IVPB medication. Now, you've been warned.

Where's The Action?

Ask to observe procedures that commonly happen on your floor and other units. Take notes during procedures. These will become golden when you're alone.

Slow Confidence

Slow down. Take your time. Slow and steady looks more like relaxed confidence, fast and hurried looks dangerous and nervous.

Wipe and Flush

Always wipe your ports with alcohol and flush your PIVs with normal saline before using them. Always!

It's in the Book

Use your handbook for clinical skills. You can read over the skills that are ordered by your patient's doctor. Also, keep your nursing textbooks. You can use these as references throughout your first few years of nursing.

Learn

Learn from your mistakes and the mistakes of others. If there is an enormous mistake made on the floor or within the hospital, take notes, and find out how to prevent this mistake from happening to you and your patient.

I Can't Come to Work

In nursing, you make your schedule through self-scheduling. Self-scheduling requires you to request the days you want to work. If you cannot come to work on the day that you are scheduled, you can call-in. Use your resources to find out the call-in and self-scheduling process before you need to call-in or self-schedule.

Scheduled Procedure

Call the procedural department in the morning for the estimated time of your patient's procedure. This is outstanding information to know. You should communicate this information to the patient, but always make sure to add the disclaimer that, "the department can call for the patient earlier or later than the estimated time of the procedure.

Shoes

Wear comfortable shoes, not stylish shoes. Later on, you can probably find a combination of the two.

Mood and RN Self-Awareness

Be prepared to provide care to your assigned patients in various patient environments. Having 5-6 patients with a range of illnesses, you may have a patient who is terminally ill while caring for a patient who has just received the greatest news regarding their test results. Always keep an even demeanor. Never let your emotions get too high or too low. If you are struggling with prolonged depression or anxiety, remember that your hospital may have free counseling services. Ask your manager about their Employee Assistance Programs.

Attitude

Your attitude is the most important tool you have to overcome the terrible days and negative people. Negative people will be your çolleagues, patients, the family of patients, doctors, phlebotomists, managers, supervisors; you name them. No position is an exception. Some people cannot control their attitudes, but don't let these people control yours. Smile and move on, unless there is a need for a more in-depth conversation with this person. Your attitude is contagious. Be the light in the darkness.

Caution Wet Floors!

Housekeeping will mop floors throughout your shift, so be mindful that you should always tread lightly on wet floors. Patients aren't the only people who fall in the hospital.

Another Question?

Your patients will press you with questions and forget the very questions they have been so eager to ask. If you have a patient who is asking many questions, it's a noble idea to have your patient write down their questions to ask when the doctor rounds. You can even write keywords for their questions on the whiteboards as a conversation starter for your patient and their doctor.

The Order of Escalation

Escalate your concerns the proper way. If you have a concern with a patient or anyone while you are working on the floor, there is a chain of command. Use your **Figuring It Out** skills to identify the proper chain of command for your hospital.

Here's an example of the common titles in a hospital's chain of command:

- Charge Nurse
- Unit Supervisor / House Supervisor
- Unit Manager
- Director of Nursing

Your charge nurse and house supervisor will usually be able to solve your problems. They are usually very knowledgeable and familiar with hospital policy.

All the Great Nurses Do This

Change your patient's bed and linens while you wait for them to come back from a procedure or the bathroom. You can also politely ask the patient care tech to do so before they return to bed. Unless otherwise told, linens can be changed every other day. If a patient is requesting a daily linen change, this is a reasonable and easy request.

Calling About Patient "_______"

Never use a patient's name when communicating with other healthcare colleagues on a non-secure network. (Especially a device audible to people other than the person you are communicating with.) Doing so could violate HIPAA. Use the patient's room number.

Do This on Your Days Off

Be sure to do whatever you do to relax on your days off. Also, make a goal of consistently looking over your notes from work. You can rewrite, type, and merge multiple documents during this time. Even if it's only for a few minutes, I would designate no longer than an hour for this task. This is the way you prepare for your upcoming test. Except your test will not be on a computer or a sheet of paper. Your test will be a task that you and your preceptor have to complete.

Trash

Take funky trash out. Don't allow soiled and odorous materials to sit in your patient's trash cans. This is a straightforward solution that many nurses overlook. Housekeeping usually leaves an extra trash bag in the trash cans. If not, ask where you can find a trash bag.

I Have a Bad Assignment

Don't take your bad assignment personally unless you know without a doubt that it is personal. Speak up if you feel your assignment was too difficult. There will be occasions when the charge nurse assigns you multiple patients who should not be given to the same nurse. Ideally, your patient assignment should be balanced. You should have a mix of low and high acuity patients in your assigned group.

Patient acuity can be defined as the amount of time and assistance needed by your patient to receive quality patient care. The more of your time your patient requires, the higher their acuity. You should not have multiple high acuity patients in your group unless all nurses on your floor have multiple high acuity patients in their assigned group. Hold your ground when speaking up. Don't make a habit of this but voice your concerns so this doesn't become a regular occurrence. Never make a huge scene with your charge nurse. Pull them to the side and speak to them in private. Strategize and think through your resources if this becomes routine.

Sorry We're Short Today

It's only a matter of time before you are scheduled to work on a day when you are short-staffed. This usually happens when there aren't enough nurses scheduled to work compared to the number of patients on the unit. On this day, you will be assigned more patients than you usually are assigned to. Don't panic. Get your day started earlier than normal. Remember who and where your resources are that will best assist you with clustering your care. Start the day by completing one task and then another and then another. Continue to work smarter and not harder by utilizing your **Figuring It Out** and **Thinking Forward** skills.

The Best Medicine

Sometimes an enjoyable conversation is better than medicine. Take the time to listen to your patients and coworkers' stories. We all have arrived at our destinations through different roads. This is the one thing I enjoy on the floor more than most. You'll be surprised to learn the level of greatness found in people and their cultures. It's amazing!

Discharging and Transferring Your Patient

Ask your preceptor to go through the usual steps to discharge and transfer a patient from your unit. Write it all down. When the opportunity to discharge or transfer your patient arises, complete this task using your notes. Ask your preceptor to be on standby to be sure you're doing what's expected.

There's Value in Innovation

I can promise you that someone is complaining right now on every Med-Surg floor around the globe. Innovative ideas are lacking on the majority of Med-Surg floors. Now, you are aware that you as a Med-Surg RN PRO can bridge the gap for your floor. Think of one thing you wouldn't mind doing for the floor (i.e. cooking, crafting, organizing the unit, organizing socials or events, volunteering for a new hospital initiative, etc.). Find ways you can make life easier for your manager, and you will be a prized gem.

Are My Results Back?

Never discuss the results of procedures with a patient when you know the outcome. Good or bad, this is a rookie mistake. Let the MD communicate this information. There is an exception to the rule when the results are good, but the patient deserves at least a phone call from the doctor explaining the results.

Slow Means Slow

Push intravenous (IV) meds slowly unless there is an order not to do so. If you can't find the specific time you should give the medication over, you should call your hospital's department who specializes in medications. (Hint: this department starts with the letter "P"). If there isn't a specific time recommendation from the medication's manufacturer or your hospital pharmacy, to be safe, push the medication over 5 minutes.

Say No

Learn to say No. (i.e. "I can't do that right now, I'm busy doing _____. Can I check back in with you a little later?")

Leaders

Learn who the leaders on the floor are. There will be people on the floor who other nurses look to for advice. Find out who these individuals are. Some will be your charge nurse, and some will not have an official title but have the wisdom you need. Find them and build an authentic relationship with them. Ask for advice when you need to.

You Have 1 Hour

At most facilities, you can give medications 30 minutes to 1 hour prior, and 30 minutes to 1 hour after the time your medications are due. Use this to your advantage. Make an honest effort to give all time-sensitive medications at their due times.

Critical Labs

At some point in your orientation, you'll get a call from the lab regarding a critical lab for one of your patients. Get to a computer and open your patient's chart. Take the lab result from the person and don't forget to read back the lab value to the person. Chart the lab value and immediately page the MD. At most facilities critical labs need to be documented the minute you find out about them.

Solo

When your preceptor gives you more time alone with your patients, you may start to feel you are alone. Remind yourself that you have an entire team there to ask questions. It may seem that you are on your own, but you are never alone.

Know Thyself

You should take the time to learn yourself and the positions you want to pursue in your career. Time will fly, and before you know it, you will be five years into nursing and feeling the pressure of burnout. Do not let this be the case. You can prevent this by creating a vision, then pursuing your vision one shift at a time. Many Med-Surg nurses are stuck at the bedside and, as a result, have poor attitudes about their work and their patients. This brings down the morale of the specialty. It makes it extremely difficult to come to work. These are the people who disrupt the unit. Stay away from these nurses early in your nursing career. The average Med-Surg workday is demanding; the least we can do is preserve the best qualities in people so we can laugh and have a great time at work. The Med-Surg RN PRO protects the Med-Surg work environment from negativity because all Med-Surg nurses deserve a work environment that is challenging yet a pleasure to work in. Find out who you are and write out your vision for your life and career. Use Med-Surg nursing as a stepping stone in pursuing your vision.

You Are Always Right

You are always right when you do what's best for the patient. Do not do what's best for you, the nurse manager, or what's best for the doctors. Do what is best for the patient.

Speak Up

You must speak up for those who cannot speak up for themselves. These are usually your less educated or English as a second language patients. As a Med-Surg RN PRO, it is your duty and privilege to guarantee that these patients receive a high level of care by using your **Thinking Forward** and **Figuring It Out** skills. You just may increase their confidence in the healthcare system that could one day save their lives.

Patient Education

Print out information for the patient who is curious and borderline apprehensive about their care. They will appreciate your thoughtfulness. Use your **Figuring It Out** skills to locate where the hospital approved patient education is located. This could be a receipt for patient education if your patient denies being educated on a medication, procedure, etc.

Patient Leaving the Floor

When the patient transporter arrives to take your patient for a procedure:

1. Be sure your patient is stable enough to go for the procedure. (If your patient is unstable, most procedural areas will require the RN to come down with the patient.) Be sure your patient will be

connected to wall oxygen as soon as they arrive at their destination.
2. Recall why and where your patient is going.

If a patient is returning to their room via a patient transporter, make a beeline to their room and lay eyes on them to make sure they are alive and well. The most common mistake I've seen in these situations is oxygen connected to an empty portable oxygen tank. Portable oxygen tanks do not last long. If you have a patient on oxygen, be sure to reconnect your patient back to the wall oxygen supply. Also, make sure the bed and call light are plugged into the wall outlet. Restart their continuous IV fluids, reset bed alarm, and reconnect Sequential Compression Devices (SCDs) if applicable.

Do the Unexpected

Be helpful to other nurses. Offer to turn patients or check on a call light that is alarming. Never help a patient out of bed or do anything unless you are confident in performing the tasks.

Wait Just a Minute

Never get another nurse's patient out of bed without the primary nurse's permission. Call the nurse while you're at the patient's bedside and ask if it is okay to get their patient out of bed.

Be On IV Watch

Watch as many IV starts as you can. You want to pull your weight and be confident in starting your own IVs.

Check and Recheck

Recheck your vital signs if the most recent set isn't consistent with prior vitals taken. Compare and be safe.

The Phone Call Trap

Family and friends of patients will call you asking for updates on their family members. Do not give any information to the person until your patient has confirmed that it is okay to speak about their healthcare with this person. You cannot speak about your patient's Protected Health Information (PHI) without your patient's consent. Doing so would violate the Health Insurance Portability and Accountability Act (HIPAA). You may be able to find the consented person's name in your patient's emergency contact section of their electronic chart. Do not forget to chart that verbal permission was given if that was the case. (Include the family member's full name and relationship in your documentation.)

Your patient and their family should decide who will be the designated contact to receive updates regarding your patient's care. Do not provide an update to everyone who calls or comes by to visit your patient.

Think Forward and consider the questions your patient's family member may have based on your patient's diagnoses and past or future tests or procedures. It is okay to refer to your **MSRNPRO** report sheet or to say, "Let me open their electronic medical chart so I can give you the most recent information we have."

Quicker Nurse Notes

Find out how to use smart text for your nursing notes. Smart text is a short phrase that you can enter a patient's chart that will expand into a pre-typed phrase that you can create for all phrases you routinely enter in your patients' nursing notes.

Plan for a Break

Plan your morning, early in the morning. We overestimate what we can do in a brief period and underestimate what we can do over a long period. Choose your morning break time. Next, consider your ideal lunch break time. Then, plan what your day will look like after 3 pm.

Snacks

Remember to bring something that can be a quick snack for those occasions that you can't eat at your usual break time. If you do, you will have a snack that you can eat in a few minutes and then get back to work until you can take your official break.

Check-in with the Charge Nurse

Always communicate clinical changes in your patients with your charge nurse. Here's an example of doing so:

> *"Hey (charge nurse's name), I just wanted to let you know my patient in room 213 is showing signs of a stroke. We are checking his vital signs now and I paged the provider. I'm headed back to his room. Would you like to come to look at him with me?"*

Look Through My Bag

Never search through a patient's belongings. There could be needles or the most disgusting object you can think of in their bags. If a patient asks you to search through their bag, kindly hand the bag to the patient. Allow the patient time to search through the bag themselves and then return the bag to the previous location.

Are You Qualified?

Occasionally a doctor or surgeon will perform a quick invasive procedure at the bedside. For example, an incision and drainage of an abscess. In this situation, you should review your hospital's policy regarding bedside procedures and check with your charge nurse regarding the necessary steps for performing a bedside procedure.

For starters, the doctor should:

1. Have the right to perform the procedure at your facility.
2. Have a signed consent from the patient specifically for the procedure.
3. Perform a "time out" before the procedure.

Why? There have been occasions when doctors quickly come by to request supplies from the nurse to perform a procedure, only to later find out that the doctor was a resident who should have been accompanied by an Attending Physician or a surgeon and did not have the right to perform procedures at that particular hospital. You shouldn't allow a random doctor the freedom to perform a procedure on your patient. Who's to say this person is even a credentialed doctor if they have not completed the process to perform a procedure at your facility.

Can This Patient Transfer to a Higher Level of Care?

Don't be afraid to ask the assigned doctor if they can move your patient to a higher level of care when the patient is clinically getting worse. Listening to the morning report, you may be able to tell if the patient needs to transfer to a higher level of care. I've cared for patients who were becoming sicker as the shift progressed, and the doctor waited until the end of the shift to transfer the patient. This isn't a good thing. It will wear you out. You will probably receive new orders every hour to address the patient's declining clinical picture. Your patient's care will be somewhat delayed because the patient could have been moved sooner. These patients will be better cared for in this situation. The fact of the matter is you only have so much time to spend with each patient on a Med-Surg unit. Sicker patients require faster and more frequent interactions. You will more than likely be behind or drowning in tasks for your other patients when you intentionally keep a sick patient that can be transferred to a higher level of care.

Your Lifeline

Your case manager or social worker will be your lifeline. They are the experts at finding community resources for your patients. Med-Surg patients have a variety of social needs that we can't fix. Your case manager can make their life easier. If your patient has a need that pulls on your heartstrings, they are a candidate to be seen by your case manager. Reach out to the case manager to explain your patient's situation and ask if they could stop by to briefly speak with the patient (Social needs, i.e. homeless, abusive relationships, loss of employment, drug abuse, emotional instability, etc.).

Bless em'

If you notice that a patient or family member is emotional, reach out to your chaplain and request a visit for prayer for your patient. This is also a marvelous idea if you have a patient who you think would enjoy a great conversation. The chaplain can pray and will usually have the time that you do not have to converse with your patient. Most times, people only want someone to listen.

Don't Sleep Around

I know this may seem to be a given, but I guess some people don't understand. Healthcare is a small community. You do not want to be the talk of a hospital or a unit for any reason other than you are a pleasure to work with.

Months 6-8

During these months, review each PRO-Tip on the PRO-Tip checklist. Place a checkmark next to the PRO-Tip that you have completed on your unit. This will help you better assess where you are in the process of entering into Med-Surg RN PRO status. Your goal should be to have at least a 90% completion of all PRO-Tips.

March through these two months using your previous months' experiences of **Thinking Forward**, **Figuring It Out**, **Task Management,** and **PRO-Tips** to become an established Med-Surg RN PRO. This is the time to work on those areas in which you want to see improvement.

*(See Appendix C to complete the PRO-TIP checklist.)

FINISHING INSIGHTFULLY STRONG

10

"Many will start fast, few will finish strong. A ferocious concentration and fanatical execution is what you need to finish strong."

Gary Ryan Blair

Months 9 and 10

You are growing more and more at this point in your journey as a Med-Surg RN PRO. Take your time to understand this brief section and the wisdom it offers.

HCAHPS- Patient Satisfaction

Hospital Consumer Assessment of Healthcare Providers and Systems started in 2006, but in 2007, hospitals that use the Inpatient Prospective Payment System (IPPS) were required to collect and submit HCAHPS data to receive their annual reimbursements. In 2010, the Affordable Care Act introduced Value-Based Purchasing, which includes HCAHPS performance to determine payment calculations for hospitals. There are nine total survey topics and nursing care effects seven.

The financial health of your hospital largely depends on HCAHPS surveys. The Centers for Medicare and Medicaid (CMS) decide financial reimbursement amounts based on the results of HCAHPS surveys that are randomly sent to recently discharged patients. These scores can be found on the internet.by individuals searching for hospitals that provide quality care. Understanding the HCAHPS allows you a better awareness of your value as a Med-Surg RN PRO.

These are the questions the HCAHPS survey will ask your patients:

- Did your nurses communicate well?
- Did you receive help as soon as you needed it?
- Was your pain well-controlled?
- How frequently did you healthcare staff explain your medications before administering them?
- How frequently were your rooms and bathrooms cleaned?
- Were the areas around your room quiet at night?
- Did you receive information about recovering at home?
- Rate the hospital on a scale of 1 to 10.

- Would you recommend the hospital?

These questions are simply a standardized data collection tool for measuring patients' perception of their hospital care. This is an attempt to create an incentive for hospitals to improve their quality of care. Why is the HCAHPS survey such a big deal to the Med-Surg RN PRO?

As a nurse, there will be times when it seems like your leaders value the opinion of your patient more than the opinion of you and your colleagues. Don't take this personally. You are now prepared to experience this reality and understand that through your Med-Surg RN PRO preparation, you are contributing to the overall financial well-being of your hospital. Your aim is to provide exceptional care through the Med-Surg RN PRO mindset. You will be more valuable to your employer than your counterpart who does not notice the financial impact of their daily patient interactions.

Finances

Pay attention to your finances. The worst people to work with in the hospital are people who are financially strapped. You feel their stress. Remember, hospitals are in the healthcare business. You, as a nurse, are in the business of caring for yourself and then others. There is no business without finances. Your finances impact your quality of life inside and outside the walls of your particular hospital.

Budget

Create a budget based on the after-tax income, your take home pay. Figure out the difference between your take-home pay and the total amount of your living expenses. Do not live outside your means. You will be a miserable wreck if you start this habit. Spend less than you earn. Take 24 hours to think through purchases greater than $250. Do not use credit cards unless you can pay off the total amount at the end of the month. Set goals for the lifestyle you want to live and do not add debt to reach your goals. Take your time with your budgeting goals. Stick to your budget. There are plenty of books, podcasts, and free videos that explain how to create a practical budget to live by.

If you want to purchase something relatively expensive, make a budget for it and slowly work towards your goal. Don't forget to add upcoming events and activities to your budget sheet. Be reasonable regarding the amount of money you set aside.

Below are a few examples of upcoming events and activities:

- Wedding
- Eating out with friends
- Saving for a house
- Saving for a dependable car
- Old and new hobbies

- Student loan payoff
- Live entertainment

Dependable Transportation

If you don't have a dependable car, this should be one of your first major purchases after you've landed your first job. I rode the city bus and train during my first six months of employment, and this was fine. If you live in an urban area, be sure to budget your transportation expenses. If owning a car makes good sense, find a dependable, budget friendly vehicle that will always have you at work on time. Don't get written up or receive corrective action because you don't have dependable transportation. It happens.

Retirement

Your employer offers a retirement plan and possibly a company match. A company match means that your employer will match the amount of money you put into your retirement plan. There are usually limits to the company match. For example, they may match up to 6% of the amount of money you put into the company's retirement account. Be sure you are enrolled in this retirement plan, at least to the amount your company will match. Immediately enroll in this plan if you haven't already. This is massively important. This is the one thing that I did not do in my first year of nursing and regret to this day. Don't be like me, reach out to your benefits department if you need instructions on how to enroll. Every day you are not enrolled is a day you miss out on the opportunity to receive free money. When you are not enrolled in your company's retirement plan, you forfeit the power you possess to allow compound interest to build wealth for you and your family.

What's compound interest? Compound interest is interest earned on money that has already earned interest. For example, if you elect to have $300 per month placed into your company retirement account that yields an 8% annual return starting at age 20 and continue to have the same amount deposited until age 60 years old, you would have more than 1 million in this account. Now if you have your employer remove this $300 from your pay and place it in your retirement account at age 30 and continue until you turn 60 years old, you would have roughly $440,445. You missed out on half a million dollars in those ten years, even though it would have been only $36,000 out of your pocket. The money put into the account will make its own money when it grows at an 8% rate. That's compound interest.

I don't think you are 20 years old, but the fundamental point is the earlier you start, the better. Send as much to your retirement account as you can, as early as you can. Also, remember that you can withdraw from these accounts in the event of an emergency. Albert Einstein said that compound interest is the most powerful force in the universe. Enroll now in your retirement plan, your family will thank you later.

Emergency Fund

Save at least $2000 for an emergency fund. If you spend any money out of this fund, replace it immediately. It's a splendid idea to move a set amount to this fund every pay period. Every time you get a raise or bonus, send an additional amount to this fund. The larger your emergency fund, the less stress you will carry. An emergency will inevitably happen. Will you be prepared?

Without a solid financial plan, you will soon find out you frequently need more money. Your first year your overall aim is the formation of a great professional foundation. Without learning the basics, it doesn't matter how much you make. What really matters is how much you keep or invest. Without consistent budgeting, you will never make enough. If you apply the recommendations from this book, in 5-10 years you'll be in an impressive financial and mental position as a nurse.

Months 11 and 12

You are probably considering what's next. You have learned a lot, and you are now a precious asset to the healthcare community. Following are a few things to consider at this point in your Med-Surg RN PRO progression.

Cross-Training

Don't stick with a job you don't like. If Med-Surg isn't your thing, consider inside and outside of the hospital's system for positions that seem to be a suitable fit for you. Don't get burned out.

Continue to grow and become more valuable to your company. Is there another department in the hospital that you have an interest in? Ask your manager to check in with the manager of that department so you can cross-train in this department.

Salary

Search until you find a manager and company that values your contributions and ideas. A great salary cannot compensate for a toxic work culture. Speaking of salary, learn to negotiate for reasonable pay. A wise person once told me that he never took the first offer. I learned this after taking the first offer twice for two previous positions. Obviously, as a new grad, you take what you can get. But after your first year and making Med Surg RN PRO status, negotiate your salary.

The best time to negotiate your salary in nursing is during the hiring process. Rarely will a nurse walk into their manager's office asking for a raise and get one. Typically, Human Resources will say your pay offer is based on years of experience. There are a few tasks that you can complete and then use as leverage to negotiate a better salary. $3-5 per hour more than the average area pay rate is a win, but you should shoot for the stars.

Your previous work should speak for itself. Make an impact on your unit that adds value to your company. Remember, healthcare is a business, and your business is looking for a return on their investment.

Here are a few tasks that will add more leverage as you negotiate your salary:

- Advanced Cardiovascular Life Support (ACLS) Certification
- Nurse Preceptor
- Cross-trained
- Med-Surg Certification
- Charge RN experience
- Committee involvement
- Innovative ideas being used at your current place of employment

If you had to choose only one, I would highly recommend you obtain one of the Med-Surg certifications as soon as possible. This will place you in another class of nurses within your specialty. A nurse with a specialty certification is one thing hospital systems love to see walking through their doors. Certifications are associated with better patient outcomes and better patient experiences.

11

ENCOURAGEMENT FORTHE MED-SURG RN PRO

"But he said to me, "My grace is sufficient for you, for my power is made perfect in weakness." Therefore, I will boast all the more gladly of my weaknesses, so that the power of Christ may rest upon me. For the sake of Christ, then, I am content with weaknesses, insults, hardships, persecutions, and calamities. For when I am weak, then I am strong."

2 Corinthians 12:9-10

I remember when I first became a Medical-Surgical nurse. My transition from nursing school to bedside nursing was a tough one. I found a job eight months after graduating from nursing school. My job title was Short-term Disability Claims Manager for AT&T. This was a non-clinical job, so you can imagine the challenges I would run into after being there for about a year. I applied for a Surgical

Intensive Care Resident position and was hired. I knew I would be expected to remember previously learned skills from my nursing school clinicals in my new position.

Throughout my three months in the Surgical Intensive Care (SICU) at Parkland Memorial Hospital, I would fail and fail hard. Every day that I pulled up to the hospital would be another very difficult shift. My preceptors were frustrated and rightfully so. Eventually, I sat down with my Nurse Manager, preceptor, and Nurse Educator to declare I needed more time to work on my time management in another area. Everyone agreed, and I had seven business days to interview for another RN position within the hospital's system. If I would've failed to find a job before the end of the seven days, I would've owed the hospital $20,000 because I signed a contract at the beginning of the Surgical Intensive Care Residency. I was later interviewed and hired to work on Parkland's Emergency General Surgical Med-Surg Unit. This is where I started my career as a Med-Surg nurse.

I was back home facing one of the hardest times of my life, but I soon remembered, it was back here in Dallas where my faith originated. My faith guided me through nursing school, where I should have failed out at least four times. I advise you to have faith in the process of becoming a Med-Surg RN PRO, faith in yourself, and faith outside of yourself. Faith is the confidence that what we hope for will actually happen. It gives us assurance about things we cannot see. In 2003, I placed my faith in the

Gospel of Jesus Christ after playing pickup basketball. This was a pivotal time in my life. I had grown up as an at-risk kid in the inner city of Dallas without many positive role models. While in high school I worked in the nutritional services department at Baylor University Medical Center in Dallas Texas. At seventeen, I was working in the basement of the hospital with ex-convicts that I had more in common with than the nursing staff I briefly interacted with when delivering food carts to the floors. It was during this time, I started to consider what I wanted to do with my life. I decided to go to college to pursue Nursing. I learned so much from my experience in the kitchen, but I wanted to explore what was taking place on those medical floors. Without my basement kitchen experience, there wouldn't be a Med-Surg RN PRO movement.

You may be wondering what about the "Gospel of Jesus Christ " led a directionless teenager to a career path that would allow him to care for men and women of every thinkable background. I would have to say, it was the undeniable grace revealed in the story of Jesus' earthly mission. Grace is defined as God's undeserved favor, which is freely available to you and me.

(**Romans 5:2-5**) Because of our faith, Christ has brought us into this place of undeserved privilege where we now stand, and we confidently and joyfully look forward to sharing God's glory. We can rejoice, too, when we run into problems and trials, for we know that they help us develop endurance and endurance develops strength of character, and character strengthens our confident hope of salvation. And this hope will not lead to disappointment. For we know how dearly God loves us, because he has given us the Holy Spirit to fill our hearts with his love.

Jesus' life mission oozed purpose and heavily reflected God's grace. We all have a unique purpose. I often remind myself, especially during the difficult moments on the floor, that it's only by the grace of God that we have the privilege of caring for patients in our communities as Med-Surg nurses. I also believe it's God's undeserved favor that allows your patients to have a nurse who has taken the time to prepare to be the best of the best within our profession.

My prayer is that your **Thinking Forward, Task Management,** and **Figuring It Out** skills will serve you well for the rest of your career. There is wisdom in the **PRO-Tips** here in this book, but they only work if you apply them to your area of practice. You are an important part of lifting the Medical-Surgical specialty out of its sometimes stagnant and underappreciated position. Always remember, you are more than capable of becoming all that you are dreaming to become.

You now have all you need to consistently approach each challenge on your assigned Med-Surg unit with the Med-Surg RN PRO mindset. Search for others who you think should explore becoming a Med-Surg RN PRO. Create a community of Med-Surg RN PROs within your community. You are part of the bright future of Medical-Surgical medicine. This material can continue to be used as a practical method of support throughout your transition from nursing school to your Medical-Surgical Unit. I am not advocating for your learning to stop after your first year on the unit. Continue to learn and build upon the skills and habits you've developed within this first year. Let your PRO Nurse Brand overflow onto those you care for with a high dose of integrity, compassion, and empathy, coupled with competent, evidence-based nursing practice. I sincerely hope you feel more professional and fearless than you ever imagined you'd be. Congratulations! You are now exactly what healthcare has been waiting for; a committed Med-Surg RN PRO!

Thanks for reading,

The Med-Surg RN PRO movement seeks to change healthcare through a nursing practice that values intentional preparation, healthy work environments, and better nurse and patient care experiences. Visit www.medsurgrnpro.com for more resources.

APPENDICES

Download free PDF copies of all of the following documents at www.medsurgrnpro.com

APPENDIX A

MSRNPRO Report Sheet

The **MSRNPRO** concept is meant to capture all of the important information about your patients. You will add your style of report taking as you grow in your routine. You may add more specifics as you build on your foundational skills. You don't have to think about how you want to group your patient information with this report sheet. You can give your end of shift report to an incoming nurse starting at the left upper column of your patient's section of the sheet (RM:) and reading down the column (columns run vertically). Continue your report at the next column starting with Hx: (patient history) and so forth until you conclude your report with Barriers to D/C. *Refer to the MSRNPRO sheet for a better understanding.

RM: Patient's room number and building, if applicable. (ex. Main building, room 623/M623)

Patient: Place a patient label here. You can cover the room number section if you have to and write the room number on the patient label. This will give you their important information. (i.e. Name, D.O.B, medical record number, etc.)

Dx: The patient's chief complaint or admitting diagnosis.

Code: Patients code status.

Aox__ Orientation and confusion should be noted here.

RA/O2 If the patient is on room air circle "RA" if the patient is on oxygen, write in how many litters.

Mobility: How does the patient walk? (i.e. up ad-lib, stand by assist with the walker, max assist, bed bound, etc.)

Hx: Patient's important medical history.

Allergies: Medication allergies.

Diet/BS: Patient diet type and Accu-check frequency if applicable.

Primary MD: Hospitalist assigned to your patient for your shift.

MD Consults: Specialty consults following your patient. (Nephrology, Cardiology, Urology, Pulmonary, Neurology, Infectious Disease, etc.)

Telemetry: If the patient is on tele, what is their Rhythm?

Calls to MD: These are the calls you will make to the doctors throughout the shift. Time/Reason: (Example: 12:30 - Patient vomiting.)

Skin: Skin breakdown.

Bowel/Bladder: How does the patient void (bowel and bladder). (Example: voids per urinal or bedside commode.)

Meds: Timely medications specific to your patient's condition.

IV: Peripheral IV location.

Fluids: Continuous fluid type and rate.

PRN Meds: Relevant PRN orders and given medications.

Labs: Relevant lab values outside of normal limits.

I&O: Intake and Output throughout a shift.

Procedures: Procedures that have been completed or need to be completed. Write the procedure type and brief results or draw a square next to the procedure type if it needs to be completed. Check the box when complete. (Example: CT Head, MRI Brain, Cardiac Catheterization, etc.)

Notes/Tasks/Goals: Your to-do list section and any information that you need to capture throughout the shift.

Barriers to D/C? What is keeping this patient in the hospital (further testing, IV antibiotics, physical therapy evaluations, long term care facility placement, etc.)?

RN I: Off-going nurse who gives you report and time of the report.

RN II: Incoming nurse who you will give report and time of report.

APPENDIX B

Things the MSRNPRO knows!

Where to find hospital policies

How to take and enter vital signs

How to page doctors

What to do if your doctor isn't answering.

Where is the tube station Codes for all locked rooms on the unit

Where to find hospital approved printable patient education

Where to get clean linens

Where to dispose of soil linen

Where to get trash bags

Where to dispose of trash

Where is the clean supply room

Where to find newly delivered medications

What is the process for patients going for procedures

How to set and turn off the bed alarm

How to answer the call light

How to connect patients to nasal cannula oxygen and how to increase oxygen amount

Where to find a portable oxygen tank

Where to place a portable oxygen tank on bed

How to tell if an oxygen tank is empty

Where to find the nasal cannula

Where to find extra vital sign machines

Where to find consents for procedures

What's the phone number to nutritional services and the phone number to the nutritional services supervisor

What's the name of your housekeeping or environmental services colleague

How to contact your Respiratory Therapist for the shift

How to contact your Case Manager for the shift

How to contact your Physical Therapist and Occupational Therapist for the shift

How to call a code blue

How to steer a bed

Who to call for a clean bed

How to set a bed's alarm

Where's the bladder scanner

How to contact your hospital chaplain

How to call security

How to apply the cardiac monitor to your patient when transferring to a higher level of care

Where to find walkers and wheelchairs

Where to find a clean SCD machine

Where to find Sani-Cloth wipes for cleaning

Where to find extra gloves

How to enter a maintenance request

Who to call for more IV pumps and poles

APPENDIX C

Med-Surg RN
PRO-Tips Checklist

- ❑ Put Out Those Fires
- ❑ Raise the Bed
- ❑ Preceptor Options
- ❑ Be as Cool as a Cucumber
- ❑ Don't Over Commit
- ❑ Change Your Gloves
- ❑ No Doubt, This Will Humble You
- ❑ Where's the Action
- ❑ Slow Confidence
- ❑ Wipe and Flush
- ❑ I Can't Come to Work
- ❑ Scheduled Procedure
- ❑ Shoes
- ❑ Mood and RN Self-Awareness
- ❑ Attitude
- ❑ Caution Wet floors!
- ❑ Another Question?
- ❑ The Order of Escalation
- ❑ All the Great Nurses Do This!

- ❑ Calling About Patient XYZ
- ❑ Do This on Your Days Off
- ❑ Trash
- ❑ I Have a Bad Assignment
- ❑ Sorry, We're Short Today
- ❑ The Best Medicine
- ❑ Discharging and Transferring Your Patient
- ❑ There's Value in Innovation
- ❑ Are My Results Back?
- ❑ Slow Means Slow
- ❑ Say No
- ❑ Leaders
- ❑ You Have 1 hour
- ❑ Critical labs
- ❑ Solo
- ❑ Know Thyself
- ❑ You're Alway Right
- ❑ Patient Education
- ❑ Patient Leaving the Floor
- ❑ Do the Unexpected
- ❑ Wait Just a Minute
- ❑ Be on IV watch
- ❑ Check and Recheck
- ❑ The Phone Trap
- ❑ Quick Nurse Notes

- ❑ Plan for a Break
- ❑ Check in with the Charge Nurse
- ❑ Look Through my Bag
- ❑ Are You Qualified
- ❑ Can This Patient Transfer?
- ❑ Your Lifeline
- ❑ Bless em'
- ❑ Don't Sleep Around

Made in the USA
Monee, IL
07 December 2025

37829530R00075